Recent Advances in

Paediatrics 27

Recent Advances in

Paediatrics 27

Ian Maconochie FRCPCH, FCEM, FRCPI, PhD
Consultant in Paediatric Accident and Emergency Medicine
St Mary's Hospital
London, UK

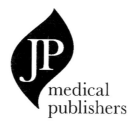

JP
medical
publishers

London • Philadelphia • Panama City • New Delhi

© 2016 JP Medical Ltd.
Published by JP Medical Ltd,
83 Victoria Street, London, SW1H 0HW, UK
Tel: +44 (0)20 3170 8910   Fax: +44 (0)20 3008 6180
Email: info@jpmedpub.com   Web: www.jpmedpub.com

ISBN: 978-1-909836-25-9

British Library Cataloguing in Publication Data
A catalogue record for this book is available from the British Library

Library of Congress Cataloging in Publication Data
A catalog record for this book is available from the Library of Congress

Commissioning Editor: Steffan Clements
Editorial Assistant: Sophie Woolven
Design: Designers Collective Ltd

Preface

The role of acting as editor in chief for the *Recent Advances in Paediatrics* series is an extremely enjoyable one. I am delighted be able to commission articles from leading experts in their fields on topics that interest those who care about the welfare of children. The topics are deliberately wide ranging and the authors have striven to highlight and comment on new areas in paediatrics. They have each written their chapter in a manner that makes those new developments in the field accessible and interesting to the general paediatric reader. The range of topics run from the establishment of the WHO course, Emergency Triage and Treatment (ETAT), and how it was set up in Africa, to rehabilitation of head injury, sports medicine in childhood, developments in paediatric intensive care, how the intranasal route may be the best mode for giving drugs in specific circumstances, the debate about immunising for RSV and more. Important practical aspects are also highlighted in the chapters, meaning that there are many learning points that can be used to improve the care of paediatric patients. I hope that you enjoy reading the contents of this volume as much as I have.

Ian Maconochie
August 2015

Contents

Chapter 1

Respiratory consequences of premature birth

Sarah J Kotecha, Sailesh Kotecha

INTRODUCTION

Preterm infants form a significant portion of total births, and the number of these infants surviving to adulthood is increasing. Current neonatal intensive care practices such as antenatal corticosteroids, gentler mechanical ventilation and postnatal surfactant have improved the long-term survival of preterm infants over recent years. On average, 10% of all worldwide births each year are preterm (<37 weeks' gestation). This translates into over 56,000 and 480,000 preterm births each year in the United Kingdom and in the United States respectively. In 2011, 7.1% of births were preterm in England and Wales [1]. Of the 7.1% of births that were preterm (<37 weeks' gestation), 5.0% were extremely preterm (<28 weeks' gestation), 11.2% were very preterm (between 28 and 31 weeks' gestation) and 83.8% were born between 32 and 36 weeks' gestation [1]. It is increasingly recognised that late preterm birth, often classified as between 32 and 36 weeks' gestation, is associated with long-term respiratory morbidity.

An understanding of the long-term respiratory consequences of premature birth is essential. Bronchopulmonary dysplasia (BPD) or chronic lung disease (CLD) of prematurity is a chronic respiratory disease which is a sequelae of preterm birth and is a consequence of perinatal and/or neonatal lung injury. BPD has been diagnosed in several ways on the basis of the need for supplemental oxygen. The most commonly used are the need for supplemental oxygen at 36 weeks postmenstrual age (PMA) or the need for supplemental oxygen for at least 28 days after birth. Our recent systematic review showed decreased lung function [forced expiratory volume in 1 second (FEV_1)] in subjects born preterm (<37 weeks' gestation), with and without BPD during childhood and beyond [2]. The mean differences [95% confidence interval (CI)] for percentage predicted FEV_1 (%FEV_1) compared with term-born controls were –7.2% (–8.7%, –5.6%) for the preterm-born group without BPD, and -18.9% (–21.1%, –16.7%) for the preterm-born group with BPD (defined as supplemental oxygen dependency until at least 36 weeks PMA). Children and adults who did not develop BPD in their infancy are at risk of long-term deficits in lung function. Children born preterm – whether they have BPD in their infancy or not – also

Sarah J Kotecha BSc SRD, Department of Child Health, Cardiff University School of Medicine, Cardiff, UK

Sailesh Kotecha PhD FRCPCH, Department of Child Health, Cardiff University School of Medicine, Cardiff, UK. Email: kotechas@cardiff.ac.uk (for correspondence)

have increased respiratory symptoms when compared with children born at term [3]. A large proportion of preterm-born school-aged children have parentally reported respiratory symptoms, such as wheeze, cough and dyspnoea, during the last 12 months.

Since lung function is thought to track throughout life, there are concerns that airway obstruction established in early childhood in this large vulnerable group of the population will lead to later development of chronic obstructive pulmonary disease. Filippone et al found that maximal flow at functional residual capacity (V_{max} FRC) measured at 2 years of age showed a significant positive correlation with lung function at a mean age of 8.8 years in children who had BPD [4]. **Figure 1.1** shows the positive correlation with lung function at the two time points.

This review will discuss the following:
1. The short- and long-term respiratory outcomes of preterm births
2. The impact of respiratory infections and atopy on respiratory consequences
3. The treatment and management of respiratory consequences of premature birth

RESPIRATORY MORBIDITY IN THE NEONATAL PERIOD

It is well documented that infants born extremely/very preterm have increased rates of admission to the neonatal intensive care unit, increased respiratory morbidity and increased health care utilisation in early life compared to term-born infants. The health care utilisation is even greater for preterm-born infants with BPD who are discharged on supplemental home oxygen [5].

In the United States, data collected retrospectively over 200,000 deliveries between 2002 and 2008 were used to compare term-born and late preterm-born subjects (34–36 weeks' gestation) for short-term respiratory morbidity. The late preterm-born infants were more

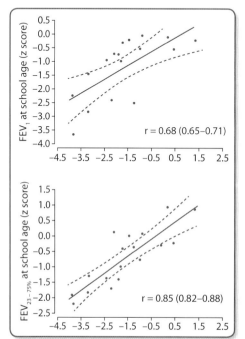

Figure 1.1 Relationship between V_{max} FRC at 24 months and postbronchodilator forced expiratory volume in 1 second and forced expiratory flow 25–75% at school age. The solid line is the regression line, and dotted lines are 95% confidence intervals. Reproduced from Filippone M, et al. [4] with permission from Elsevier.

likely to be admitted to a neonatal intensive care unit compared to the term-born infants (36.5% and 7.2% respectively). In addition, of those admitted to the neonatal intensive care unit, the late preterm-born infants were more likely to be admitted due to respiratory compromise than the term-born infants (28.8% and 15.6% of those admitted respectively). The late preterm-born infants had increased respiratory morbidity in the neonatal period compared to the term-born infants, in particular, respiratory distress syndrome, transient tachypnoea of the newborn and pneumonia [6].

EARLY INFECTION

As mentioned previously, there are many reports of increased hospitalisation and increased respiratory symptoms of preterm-born children both extremely/very preterm and moderate/late preterm. Boyce et al, in a large retrospective cohort study, estimated the number of respiratory syncytial virus (RSV) hospitalisations during the first year of life per 1000 children was 70 for children born ≤28 weeks' gestation, 66 for children born at 29 to <33 weeks, 57 for children born at 33 to <36 weeks and 388 for children with BPD, compared to 30 for children born at term without underlying medical condition [7]. However, the rates of hospitalisation due to RSV were no higher after 12 months of age for the preterm-born children compared to term-born children without underlying medical conditions who were <12 months old. A large Swedish study noted that a respiratory infection requiring hospitalisation in the first year of life is associated with an increased risk of asthma after the age of 5. The association between infection and later asthma risk was present across all the gestational groups, but the greatest association was in the most preterm-born subjects (<28 weeks' gestation) [8]. It is, therefore, clear that preterm birth is associated with increased hospitalisation.

THE SHORT- AND LONG-TERM LUNG FUNCTION OUTCOMES OF VERY/EXTREMELY PREMATURE BIRTHS

Traditionally, research studies and many reviews have focussed on respiratory outcomes of those who develop the neonatal lung disease, BPD, often also called CLD, and/or those preterm-born subjects who were born at <32 weeks' gestation. Preterm-born infants who develop BPD may require supplementary oxygen at home for several months or longer.

Chronic respiratory morbidity is a common consequence of preterm birth prior to 32 weeks' gestation, especially if the child had BPD in infancy [5]. As already stated in our recent systematic review [2], preterm-born subjects with BPD have greater deficits in lung function than preterm-born subjects without BPD. In the systematic review, we did note that %FEV_1 for the preterm-born subjects with BPD defined as supplemental oxygen dependency until at least 28 days of life may have improved over the years, but it was unclear if there was any selection bias to explain this improvement (**Figure 1.2**). There is evidence that during the first 2 years of life, lung function abnormalities are common and these may persist into school age and beyond. The EpiCure study, a large cohort study in the United Kingdom and Ireland, analysed children born at ≤25 weeks' gestation at 11 years of age and observed that 56% of survivors had abnormal spirometry when compared with controls. The lung function deficits were greater in the preterm-born children who had BPD than in the preterm-born children who did not have BPD [9]. Vrijlandt et al, in a prospective nationwide Dutch study of preterm-born subjects at <32 weeks' gestation and/

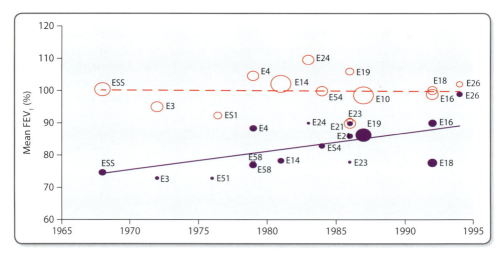

Figure 1.2 Effect of year of birth on percentage predicted forced expiratory volume in 1 second (FEV₁) for the bronchopulmonary dysplasia (BPD) group (supplemental oxygen dependency at 28 days) and the term control group. BPD group supplemental oxygen dependency at 28 days (closed circles) and the term control group (open circles). Weighting was based on two separate models, one for the BPD group and one for the term control group. Weighting was defined by variance which differs for the term control and BPD group. Bubble sizes show relative contributions based on individual weighting of term control and BPD group. The E-numbers refer to references which are given in the online data supplement. Reproduced from Kotecha SJ, et al. [2] with permission from BMJ Publishing Group Ltd.

or a birth weight under 1500 g at 19 years, noted that preterm birth was associated with lower FEV₁ and exercise capacity than term controls [10]. They did not find any significant differences in lung function or exercise capacity between the preterm-born young adults who had BPD and the preterm-born adults who did not have BPD. They conclude that 'subtle but possibly important lung function abnormalities after preterm birth may persist into adulthood.' This may have an impact in later life, since it has been shown that young adults with submaximal lung function will reach the danger zone of impaired lung function in old age more quickly [10].

THE SHORT- AND LONG-TERM LUNG FUNCTION OUTCOMES OF MODERATE/LATE PRETERM BIRTHS

Traditionally, there has been a paucity of research on the long-term outcomes of children and adults born at >32 weeks' gestation. These infants were not perceived to be at risk of short- or long-term consequences of their preterm birth. However, recently there has been much interest in this large group of the population of preterm-born survivors and an awareness that these children and adults are at risk of short- and long-term respiratory morbidity.

In one study, healthy infants born at 33–36 weeks' gestation were compared at 40 weeks PMA to healthy term infants and were noted to have altered lung function [11]. The late preterm-born infants have decreased passive respiratory system compliance and time to peak tidal expiratory flow to expiratory time; increased respiratory resistance and a higher tidal volume when compared to the term control group. These results suggest that even healthy infants born at 33–36 weeks' gestation may have abnormal or delayed pulmonary development when compared to term-born infants. Friedrich et al studied healthy infants born at 30–34 weeks' gestation in the first and second years of life and reported decreased forced expiratory flows and normal forced vital capacities [12]. Using the Avon Longitudinal Study of Parents and Children, we noted that children of 8–9 years of age born at 33–34 weeks' gestation had lower measures of forced expiratory spirometry compared to children born at term. These measures are of a similar magnitude to those observed in the extremely/very preterm (25–32 weeks' gestation) group [13]. Children born at 35–36 weeks' gestation had measures which were more similar to the term-born children. Interestingly, by 14–17 years, measures of airway function in children born at 33–34 weeks' gestation were similar to those in the term-born children with the exception of forced mid-expiratory flow between 25% and 75% of vital capacity (FEF_{25-75}; **Figure 1.3**). These data suggest that even birth at late preterm is associated with longer-term lung function deficits.

RESPIRATORY SYMPTOMS

When assessing symptoms in preterm-born children or reporting them in the medical journals, the phrase 'doctor diagnosed asthma' is frequently used, but we and others have questioned the accuracy of this phrase. Been et al conducted a systematic review and meta-analysis of preterm birth and childhood wheezing disorders using data from >1.5 million children, noting that preterm birth was associated with 1.71 times greater risk of childhood wheezing disorders compared to term-born children [an unadjusted odds ratio (OR) of 1.71 (95% CI 1.57–1.87)] [14]. When they studied very preterm born (<32 weeks' gestation), they had three times increased risk of childhood wheezing disorders compared to term-born children (an unadjusted OR of 3.00). Another systematic review and meta-analysis reported that preterm-born children have approximately 7% higher risk of asthma compared to term-born children [15]. The authors noted that the effect of prematurity on the risk of asthma decreases in later life and appeared to be strongest at a younger age. A recent article investigated if respiratory morbidity during the first year of life can be predicted by lung function tests performed at near term age (44 weeks PMA) in preterm-born infants (mean 29 weeks' gestation standard deviation ± 3 weeks' gestation). There was a significant association between tidal volume, time to peak expiratory flow/expiratory time ratio and respiratory rate with subsequent wheeze. However, when lung function was compared to standard clinical predictors, it did not improve prediction of later respiratory morbidity in individual children. They summarised that they would recommend tidal

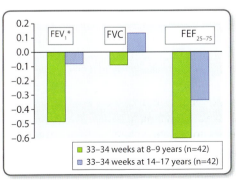

Figure 1.3 Changes in lung spirometry between 8–9 and 14–17 years for children in the Avon Longitudinal Study of Parents and Children cohort born at 33–34 weeks. FEV₁, forced expiratory volume in 1 second; FVC, forced vital capacity; FEF, forced expiratory *P<0.05. Reproduced from Kotecha SJ, et al. [13] with permission from BMJ Publishing Group Ltd.

lung function testing as a way to gain further knowledge and understanding of respiratory pathophysiology but did not recommend its use to predict respiratory symptoms during the first year of life [16]. Recent publications have also reported that late preterm-born infants and children have increased respiratory symptoms. An association between extremely preterm birth and later respiratory morbidity has been well reported previously. Boyle et al [17] in a large longitudinal study in the United Kingdom of infants born between 2000 and 2002 noted that preterm-born children born at 32–36 weeks' gestation may experience increased respiratory symptoms, often reported as asthma; have increased reported inhaled drug use and increased health utilisation, including hospitalisation, especially in early childhood. The cohort studied and hence the data are representative of the UK population. Goyal et al conducted a retrospective cohort analysis studying preterm-born infants (34–42 weeks' gestation) born in 2007. They reported that late preterm birth (34–36 completed weeks' gestation) compared to term birth (39–42 weeks' gestation) was associated with significant increases in persistent asthma diagnoses (an adjusted OR of 1.68) when they monitored children from birth to 18 months [18]. In addition, late preterm birth compared to term birth was associated with significant increases in inhaled corticosteroid use (an adjusted OR of 1.66) and the number of acute respiratory visits (an incidence rate ratio of 1.44).

ATOPY

Preterm-born children have increased wheeze often reported as increased rates of asthma. Increased atopy may explain the increased rates of reported asthma. Siltanen at al compared this incidence of atopy among 166 adults aged 18–27 years who were born preterm and at a very low birth weight ($\leq$1500 g) and 172 term-born controls [19]. They reported that the young adults who were born prematurely with a very low birth weight had a lower incidence of atopy than the controls. About 45.5% of the preterm-born adults had a positive skin prick test to at least one of the six common aeroallergens compared to 57.9% of the control group (crude OR of 0.61; 95% CI 0.39–0.93 $P = 0.023$). In a previous publication, Siltanen et al compared respiratory symptoms and lung function in relation to atopy in two groups of 10-year-old children: preterm-born children with birth weights of <1501 g and full-term children with birth weights >2500 g. Preterm-born children had more respiratory symptoms, e.g. lifetime prevalence of wheezing was 43% compared to 17% in the term-born group. However, in the term-born group, wheezing was associated with atopy, with 64% of wheezers having atopy, whereas in the preterm-born group only 23% of wheezing was associated with atopy. When lung function was measured, the preterm-born group, as in many other studies, had lower spirometry values compared to the term-born group. The lower spirometry values in the preterm-born group were associated with reported asthma, wheezing and low gestational age, but not with atopy. About 62% of children in the preterm-born group who wheezed and still wheezed at 10 years of age were atopic compared to 9% of the children in the preterm-born group who wheezed but no longer had wheezing at 10 years of age [20]. In agreement, a recent Polish publication reported that extremely low birth weight children (<1000 g) at a mean age of 6.7 years had more frequent wheezing compared to term-born children (64% compared to 25% respectively) and were diagnosed with asthma more often (32% compared to 7.5% respectively). About 60% of the extremely low birth weight children required hospitalisation ever due to respiratory problem compared to 10% of term-born children. However, the extremely low birth weight children were not different to the term-born children in the case of occurrence of allergy symptoms. The need for rehospitalisation in the first 2 years of life was an important risk factor for respiratory morbidity in the future. The need for rehospitalisation was a more important risk factor than the diagnosis of BPD or allergy and perinatal factors [21]. Atopy rates in preterm-born children are not different to term-born children, hence are unlikely to explain the increased wheezing reported in preterm-born children.

TREATMENT AND MANAGEMENT

It is apparent that there is a large population of preterm-born children and adults who have lung function deficits and respiratory symptoms which, in many cases, are underinvestigated and not treated. One can speculate that failure to institute treatment may be due to the possible absence of evidence of symptoms of 'classical' asthma including atopy in preterm-born children. In addition, the reluctance to instigate regular treatment is probably because we do not understand the underlying disease process, which, thus, needs careful evaluation to determine. In summary, the underlying mechanisms are unknown; this may lead to under or inappropriate treatment of preterm-born children with wheeze.

The EpiCure study reported that 56% of children born extremely preterm, <26 weeks' gestation, had abnormal baseline spirometry and 27% had a positive bronchodilator response, but less than half of those having lung function impairments were receiving any medication at 11 years of age [9]. Joshi et al showed marked reversible exercise-induced bronchoconstriction in preterm-born children who had BPD in their infancy at 8–12 years of age, but a few children were receiving any treatment. These children also had more respiratory symptoms than term-born controls [22]. In contrast, a large Swedish study reported over a million children aged 6–19 years and their retrieval of at least one prescription of an inhaled corticosteroid during 2006; in total 4.89% of the men and 3.78% of the women had purchased inhaled corticosteroids. They reported preterm-born children had increased inhaled corticosteroid usage. Compared to the control group – children born between 39 and 41 weeks' gestation – the OR for inhaled corticosteroid use increased with prematurity, an OR of 1.10 for children born at 37–38 weeks to 2.28 for children born between 23 and 28 weeks, this was after adjustment for confounders. The use was similar in men and women, and decreased as age increased [23A]. In another systematic review [23B] remove review and put in paper,as otherwise it reads review we have reviewed, we have reviewed the short- and long-term effect of bronchodilator administration on %FEV$_1$ in preterm-born children and adults. The studies mainly reported short-term effects after a single dose administration of a bronchodilator with a majority reporting an improvement. Disappointingly, we only found one study investigating the longer-term effects of bronchodilator administration, 2 weeks, which reported an improvement in lung function [24]. There is a paucity of date on the effect of inhaled steroid administration on the lung function of preterm-born subjects. We are aware of two studies which reported the effect of inhaled steroids on the lung function of preterm-born subjects in childhood. The inhaled steroids did not have a significant effect on spirometry [25,26] but in one study may have decreased bronchial liability [25].

There may be many reasons for the lack of treatment of the deficits in lung function observed in preterm-born children and adults. Failure to treat may be owing to the absence of evidence of 'classical' asthma symptoms including atopy in preterm-born children. Possibly, a lack of understanding of the underlying mechanism of the disease process has also impeded the management of these children and, perhaps a perception that airway obstruction in the preterm-born subjects is due to an irreversible, structural airway injury. The underlying mechanisms is likely to be either inflammatory as suggested by a study reporting neutrophilic airway inflammation [27] and increased oxidant stress assessed by measuring 8-isoprostane concentration in exhaled breath condensate [28] or due to smooth muscle hypertrophy, as suggested by pathological studies of preterm infants dying from respiratory failure.

Further research is needed to identify the underlying mechanisms of the deficits in lung function and to identify possible treatments.

CONCLUSION

In conclusion, children and adults born preterm are at risk of long-term respiratory consequences. It is not just those who are born extremely/very preterm but also those who are born late preterm have respiratory symptoms and deficits in lung function. More studies are needed particularly with regard to the children and adult who were born late preterm as they had not been studied to as greater an extent as extremely/very preterm-born children and adults. It is important to identify the mechanisms of the symptoms and the pulmonary function deficits that have been observed; and following on from this to identify specific treatments to manage the deficits in lung function and symptoms observed. Future research should focus on the causes and mechanisms of preterm-born wheeze to examine if there are any impaired lung growth or inflammatory processes taking place.

Key points for clinical practice

- An increasing number of infants are born preterm and, owing to improved medical management, are surviving to adulthood.
- Compared with term-born infants, preterm-born infants have increased respiratory morbidity, admissions to neonatal intensive care units for respiratory illnesses, and re-hospitalisation in early childhood due to respiratory illnesses compared to term-born infants.
- Very, extremely, moderate and late preterm-born subjects are at risk of long-term deficits of lung function in childhood and beyond.
- Preterm-born subjects with bronchopulmonary dysplasia may be at a greater risk of long-term respiratory consequences of prematurity than preterm-born subjects without bronchopulmonary dysplasia.
- Despite having a higher incidence of wheezing in childhood, preterm-born children do not appear in some studies to have a higher incidence of atopy than term-born children.
- It is important for adult physicians to ask about the neonatal history of their patients; however, this is currently not in common practice.
- Many preterm-born children and adults with lung function deficits do not appear to be receiving treatment but the optimal treatment/s needs to be defined.
- More research is needed particularly to understand the mechanisms of the respiratory consequences of preterm birth in extremely and late preterm-born infants.
- More research is also needed to examine longitudinal lung function outcomes and respiratory symptoms into middle age and beyond.

REFERENCES

1. Office for National Statistics (ONS). Gestation-specific infant mortality in England and Wales, 2011. Cardiff: ONS, 2013.
2. Kotecha SJ, Edwards MO, Watkins WJ, et al. Effect of preterm birth on later FEV1: a systematic review and meta-analysis. Thorax 2013; 68:760–766.
3. Vrijlandt EJ, Boezen HM, Gerritsen J, et al. Respiratory health in prematurely born preschool children with and without bronchopulmonary dysplasia. J Pediatr 2007; 150:256–261.
4. Filippone M, Sartor M, Zacchello F, et al. Flow limitation in infants with bronchopulmonary dysplasia and respiratory function at school age. Lancet 2003; 361:753–754.
5. Greenough A. Long-term respiratory consequences of premature birth at less than 32 weeks of gestation. Early Hum Dev 2013; 89:S25–S27.
6. The Consortium on Safe Labour, Hibbard JU, Wilkins I, et al. Respiratory Morbidity in Late Preterm Births. JAMA 2010; 304:419–425.
7. Boyce TG, Mellen BG, Mitchel EF, et al. Rates of hospitalization for respiratory syncytial virus infection among children in Medicaid. J Pediatr 2000; 137:865–870.
8. Montgomery S, Bahmanyar S, Brus O, et al. Respiratory infections in preterm infants and subsequent asthma: a cohort study. BMJ Open 2013; 3:e004034.
9. Fawke J, Lum S, Kirkby J, et al. Lung function and respiratory symptoms at 11 years in children born extremely preterm. The EPICure Study. Am J Respir Crit Care Med 2010; 182:237–245.
10. Vrijlandt EJ, Gerritsen J, Boezen HM, et al. Lung function and exercise capacity in young adults born prematurely. Am J Respir Crit Care Med 2006; 173:890–896.
11. McEvoy C, Venigalla S, Schilling D, et al. Respiratory function in healthy late preterm infants delivered at 33-36 weeks of gestation. J Pediatr 2013; 162:464–469.
12. Friedrich L, Pitrez PMC, Stein RT, et al. Growth rate of lung function in healthy preterm infants. Am J Respir Crit Care Med 2007; 176:1269–1273.
13. Kotecha SJ, Watkins WJ, Paranjothy S, et al. Effect of late preterm birth on longitudinal lung spirometry in school age children and adolescents. Thorax 2012; 67:54–61.
14. Been JV, Lugtenberg MJ, Smets E, et al. Preterm birth and childhood wheezing disorders: a systematic review and meta-analysis. PLoS Med 2014; 11:e001596.
15. Jaakkola JJK, Ahmed P, Leromnimon A, et al. Preterm delivery and asthma: a systematic review and meta-analysis. J Allergy Clin Immunol 2008; 118:823–830.
16. Proietti E, Riedel T, Fuchs O, et al. Can infant lung function predict respiratory morbidity during the first year of life in preterm infants? Eur Respir J 2014; 43:1642–1651.
17. Boyle EM, Poulsen G, Field DJ, et al. Effects of gestational age at birth on health outcomes at 3 and 5 years of age: population based cohort study. BMJ 2012; 344:e896.
18. Goyal NK, Fiks AG, Lorch SA. Association of late-preterm birth with asthma in young children: practice-based study. Pediatrics 2011; 128:e830.
19. Siltanen M, Wehkalampi K, Hovi P, et al. Preterm birth reduces the incidence of atopy in adulthood. J Allergy Clin Immunol 2011; 127:935–942.
20. Siltanen M, Savilahti E, Pohjavouri M, et al. Respiratory symptoms and lung function in relation to atopy in children born preterm. Pediatr Pulmonol 2004; 37:43–49.
21. Kwinta P, Lis G, Klimek M, et al. The prevalence and risk factors of allergic and respiratory symptoms in a regional cohort of extremely low birth weight children (<1000 g). Ital J Pediatr 2013; 39:4.
22. Joshi S, Powell T, Watkins WJ, et al. Exercise-induced bronchoconstriction in school-aged children who had chronic lung disease in infancy. J Pediatr 2013; 162:813–818.
23A. Vogt H, Lindstrom K, Braback L, et al. Preterm birth and inhaled corticosteroid use in 6- to 19-year-olds: a Swedish national cohort study. Pediatrics 2011; 127:1052–1059.
23B. Kotecha SJ, Edwards MO, Watkins WJ, et al. Effect of bronchodilators on forced expiratory volume in 1 s in preterm-born participants aged 5 and over: a systematic review. Neonatology 2015;107:231-240.
24. Pelkonen AS, Hakulinen AL, Turpeinen M. Bronchial lability and responsiveness in school children born very preterm. Am J Respir Crit Care Med 1997; 156:1178–1184.
25. Pelkonen AS, Hakulinen AL, Hallman M, et al. Effect of inhaled budenoside therapy on lung function in schoolchildren born preterm. Respir Med 2002; 95:565–570.

26. Chan KN, Silverman M. Increased airway responsiveness in children of low birth weight at school age: effect of topical corticosteroids. Arch Dis Child 1993; 69:120–124.
27. Teig N, Allali M, Rieger C, et al. Inflammatory markers in induced sputum of school children born before 32 completed weeks of gestation. J Pediatr 2012; 161:1085–1090.
28. Filippone M, Bonetto G, Corradi M, et al. Evidence of unexpected oxidative stress in airways of adolescents born very pre-term. Eur Respir J 2012; 40:1253–1259.

Chapter 2

Developmental dysplasia of the hips

Sami Al-Ali, Deborah M Eastwood

INTRODUCTION

Developmental dysplasia of the hips (DDH) describes a continuum of hip pathology present both in the neonate and in the child that ranges from the slightly shallow acetabulum with potentially unstable movement through to more significant hip instability and subluxation, and on to frank dislocation of the femoral head which may or may not be reducible. Klisic introduced the term DDH to replace the previous label of 'congenital dislocation of the hip' to reflect our improved understanding of the pathophysiology and the realisation that only a few cases were frank dislocations at birth [1]. Most cases of hip dysplasia involved more subtle subluxation with unstable movement preventing the normal maturation of the infant acetabulum with worsening subluxation and dysplasia: thus any individual case of DDH may progress from mild dysplasia with clinically undetectable instability at birth to a dislocated hip.

Early detection and simple treatment with a harness that facilitates concentric reduction and encourages stable movement almost invariably leads to a 'normalisation' of anatomy with remodelling of acetabular dysplasia. Unfortunately, a significant number of cases continue to be identified late necessitating more challenging interventions including surgery of significant magnitude with much higher risk and less favourable outcome. Residual dysplasia and subluxation at skeletal maturity can lead to the early onset of osteoarthritis with increasing pain and limitation of activity in early adult life necessitating joint replacement surgery. A hip replacement in a patient's 30s and 40s will inevitably fail within 15–20 years meaning a revision procedure with higher associated risks may be necessary in the 50s and 60s. It is reported that DDH accounts for 10% of all primary hip arthroplasty and 30% of those performed in the under 60s [2]. For those with more minor degrees of dysplasia at skeletal maturity, excessive point loading of the outer edge of the acetabulum and its labrum can lead to painful tears and associated morbidity, and a new subspecialty has arisen in orthopaedics to deal with such problems in the young adult hip.

Our first challenge as a professional body must be to improve our early detection of DDH or hip instability so that early treatment can be instigated when appropriate. Subsequent

Sami Al-Ali BM MRCS FRCS, The Catterall Unit, Royal National Orthopaedic Hospital, Middlesex, UK

Deborah M Eastwood FRCS, The Catterall Unit, Royal National Orthopaedic Hospital, Middlesex, UK. Email: d.m.eastwood@ btinternet.com (for correspondence)

challenges involve recognition of whether the treatment has stabilised the hip, how to monitor these patients after treatment and for how long, and how to recognise residual dysplasia and decide when, how and if to intervene. This review will outline how the paediatric orthopaedic teams are tackling these challenges. Hip dysplasia in the context of neurological injury or as part of a more complicated syndrome or skeletal dysplasia is beyond the scope of this chapter.

AETIOLOGY AND RISK FACTORS

The aetiology remains unknown but is likely to be multifactorial. Hormonal factors probably influence the female predominance of 5:1 but there has been no demonstrated association with umbilical cord relaxin or oestrogen levels and DDH [3,4]. There is a 'genetic susceptibility' to DDH with a positive family history of one or more first-degree relatives or two or more second-degree relatives constituting a significantly increased risk. There is a strong maternal effect with a higher prevalence for offspring of mothers compared to fathers or siblings [5]. As yet, no specific gene has been identified but concordance is higher with monozygotic (33%) than dizygotic twins (8%) [6].

DDH is associated with 'packaging' disorders where there is little space in the uterus (**Table 2.1**).

The left hip is more commonly affected owing to the adducted position of the left leg in utero as the baby presents in the left occipitoanterior position for delivery. Tight packaging after birth with swaddling of infants with the hips both extended and adducted contributes to an increased incidence of DDH in certain populations [4]. This detrimental effect was recognised in Japan where a nationwide programme instigated to educate and discourage swaddling led to a five-fold decrease in incidence of DDH [7]. Swaddling garments that allow the legs more freedom to move into abduction and flexion are recommended by the International Hip Dysplasia Institute (www.hipdysplasia.org).

Breech presentation is a major independent risk factor even though twice as many females are born breech. The greatest risk is for those who are breech and delivered vaginally; the risk decreases with an elective caesarean section. A breech position at any stage in the last trimester will also increase the infants' risk for DDH.

PREVALENCE

The reported incidence varies widely between countries and populations and depends heavily on the means and/or criteria used for diagnosis. In populations with a high uptake

Table 2.1 Associations with in utero tight 'packaging'	
Conditions associated with tight packaging	First pregnancy
	Oligohydramnios
	Birth weight >5 kg
	Multiple pregnancies
Other clinical features of packaging disorders	Foot deformities
	Plagiocephaly and torticollis
Postnatal packaging	Swaddling with hips extended

of ultrasound assessment, the reported rate of dysplasia will be higher, though many would go on to normalise. The lowest incidence is reported in unscreened populations reporting a prevalence of 0.8–1.6 per 1000 [8]. With clinically screened populations, the prevalence was generally higher but with significant variability: 1.6–28.5 per 1000 [8]. If the screening includes ultrasound or radiographic assessment, rates vary depending on how the parameters are defined, but are much higher: 34–60.3 per 1000. About 20% of cases have bilateral hip involvement, and this group is more likely to be diagnosed late.

PATHOPHYSIOLOGY

The hip begins to form around the seventh week of gestation. By week 11, the spherical femoral head, its matching acetabulum and the ligamentum teres are identifiable. The hip is most lax and shallow in late pregnancy to facilitate delivery [9]. The growth potential of the infant and the modelling capacity of the largely cartilaginous acetabulum are both high.

There is a significant degree of joint laxity at birth and some clinical instability is relatively common; much of this will resolve spontaneously within the first 1–3 weeks of life. Similarly, many hips identified as dysplastic soon after birth with ultrasound will normalise over the first 3 weeks without intervention. Despite this trend, many clinicians feel that any clinical or sonographic concern should be taken seriously and observed in the appropriate setting by those with the appropriate specialist interest and insight.

While preterm infants may have more laxity and are 'behind' in their normal development, they do not have a higher incidence of DDH. This may be explained in part because the term infant has the greatest laxity and is more 'tightly packed' in the late stages than its preterm counterpart.

For neonates who demonstrate instability or where excessive pressure is concentrated on part of the acetabulum, distortion of anatomy and failure of uniform growth can occur.

An unstable hip with a dysplastic (shallow) acetabulum detected early in the first few weeks of life which is concentrically reduced, and in which stable movement is facilitated, should respond well to the more physiological forces applied to it and, in the majority of cases, a normal hip will result.

DIAGNOSIS

DDH is diagnosed either early or late; there is no agreed cut-off between the two which makes it difficult to compare many studies that discuss incidence, treatment and outcomes. For the neonate and nonambulant infant, DDH is asymptomatic and its detection must be a proactive process.

History

In the context of early detection, the useful history is confined to the detection of risk factors as outlined above. Particular attention should be paid to family history and full obstetric history.

In the older infant, the family may notice 'stiff hips' when changing a nappy and there may be signs noticeable in the walking infant such as a limp or a waddle, a short leg and a tendency to tip toe. Parental concerns should always be taken seriously. Although DDH does not usually hamper the infants from taking to their feet, 20% of children with DDH will not have stood or walked by 18 months compared to 5% of children without [10].

The description of a 'clicky' hip should be taken seriously but it is not synonymous with DDH and frequently arises from iliopsoas anteriorly or fascia lata laterally clicking over the greater trochanter rather than the dislocation/reduction of a hip. Pain is not a presenting feature in childhood.

Clinical examination

In the neonate

Clinical examination of the neonate is a difficult skill to master. The environment and the hands must be warm and the baby relaxed, perhaps after a feed. The nappy must also be removed fully during a hip assessment. A general assessment of the baby is required to ensure a syndromic cause for any associated hip problems is excluded.

In the UK, it is a legal requirement that all neonates are examined and the hip assessment is an integral part of this examination. Too often, this task falls to an inexperienced member of a clinical team who is more likely to miss the clinical signs; the clinical examination should answer three questions as given in **Table 2.2**.

Inspection, with the nappy removed, may reveal a leg length discrepancy with the legs lying in extension. Asymmetrical skin creases in the groin do have an association (not absolute) with DDH; those more distally do not.

The Ortolani and Barlow [11] tests are a major part of the neonatal hip examination. While both have a high specificity of 100%, they have a low sensitivity of 60% [12] which drops significantly in inexperienced hands. Both are conducted with the hips flexed to 90° and with both knees held gently within the examiner's first web space; the fingers lie over the greater trochanter and the thumb over the medial proximal thigh. In this positon, one thigh may feel shorter than the other (Galeazzi sign positive).

The hips are then abducted in >90° of flexion; if there is any unilateral or bilateral limitation of abduction, a dislocated hip(s) must be suspected. The Ortolani test attempts to reduce a dislocated hip as the middle finger lying over the greater trochanter lifts the femoral head back into the acetabulum. This relocation of the femoral head may be very subtle and may happen inadvertently with the initial movement of the leg into abduction: as the hip abducts fully, a 'hiccough' or momentary catch is felt during the movement as the hip reduces. This test must be done gently.

If the hip is not clinically dislocated, it may be dislocatable; the legs are returned to the midline and the Barlow test is performed. This test seeks to dislocate an unstable hip by

Table 2.2 Clinical examination: the thought process	
Clinical question	Answer
Is the hip dislocated clinically? Is it reducible?	Yes, dislocated hip Yes, Ortolani positive No, Ortolani negative
If the hip is not dislocated, is it dislocatable?	Yes, dislocatable hip, Barlow positive
If the hip is not dislocated or dislocatable, is it clinically normal? Are there any risk factors?	Yes, clinically normal hip The hip may still be at risk of DDH and warrant further investigation
DDH, developmental dysplasia of the hips.	

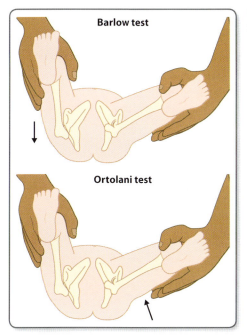

Figure 2.1 The Barlow and the Ortolani test. Arrows show the direction of force applied.

adducting the flexed hip and applying a front-to-back pressure. The Barlow test must be done gently.

Excessive force must not be applied to the vulnerable and immature femoral head. If the examination suggests the hip is clinically stable, this finding must be taken in conjunction with the history to decide whether or not the hip is still 'at risk' of DDH.

In the infant, it is important to distinguish between a 'Barlow positive hip', which is reduced at rest but unstable, and an 'Ortolani positive hip', which is dislocated at rest but reducible (**Figure 2.1**).

Both the Ortolani and Barlow tests become less sensitive after the neonatal period as the infant grows and muscle tone increases: a positive test in a child over 3 months of age should raise concerns of abnormal muscle tone and/or an underlying neurological problem.

In the infant

Limitation of hip abduction in >90° of flexion is a useful sign of DDH particularly after the age of 8 months with lower sensitivity before that age [13]. False negatives will occur if the pelvis is allowed to rock as each hip is abducted. A limitation of abduction is also less easy to detect if the hip is not flexed sufficiently. An asymmetry in movement is easier to detect than a symmetrical limitation that accompanies bilateral hip dislocation; clinicians are trained to detect asymmetry, but should be aware of 'bilateral asymmetry'.

Particularly with bilateral pathology, the perineum may seem 'wide' as both thighs have been effectively displaced laterally. The femoral head(s) may be palpable in the buttock.

While many of these signs are subtle, they are there to be elicited and any clinical concern from the history or examination should prompt the use of imaging to answer the question: is this a case of DDH or not?

Imaging

Ultrasound

The ultrasound scan (USS) is the investigation of choice for the infant hip under 4 months of age. Graf popularised the static assessment of the dysplastic hip using USS to provide a morphological description of the cartilaginous hip (prior to the onset of femoral head ossification). He defined measurements taken from a standardised view with the line of the iliac wing denoting the axis from which the α angle of the acetabular bony roof and the β angle of the cartilage roof are measured. The acetabular rim might be flat or rounded, and the femoral head may be in or out of joint. He initially categorised hips into four grades but many of these now have subtypes (**Figure 2.2** and **Table 2.3**).

The Morin index allows a snapshot assessment to be made of whether the hip is adequately seated within its acetabulum or not. However, this emphasises again the concept of hip instability, a hip that is in joint one moment and may be out the next moment. Thus, the original static USS assessment has been broadened to include a useful dynamic assessment of stability [14].

USS can be repeated regularly without irradiation and may be used to monitor improved hip development, be it spontaneous or in response to treatment (**Figure 2.3**). It has the disadvantage that it is operator dependent.

Radiographs

Radiographs are generally a more useful imaging modality after the age of 4–5 months. The hip is still largely cartilaginous at this stage and the femoral head ossification which is taken as a sign of hip maturity and stability may not be visible until 5–6 months. Its appearance is often considerably delayed in DDH and there will be an asymmetry in size in unilateral cases.

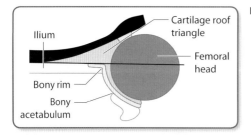

Figure 2.2 Interpretation of ultrasound.

Table 2.3 Simplified Graf classification		
Graf type	**α angle (bony roof) (degrees)**	**Bony rim**
I	>60	Angular
IIa physiologically immature	50–59	Rounded
IIb delayed ossification	50–59	Rounded
IIc	43–49	Rounded
III eccentric	<43	Flattened
IV eccentric	<43	Flattened

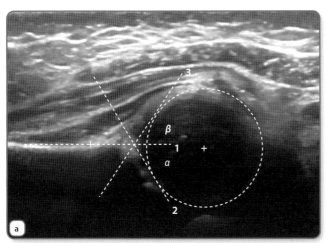

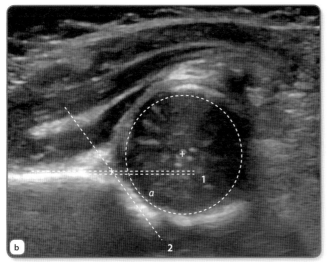

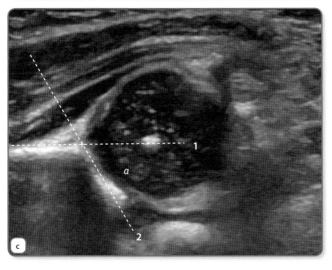

Figure 2.3 (a) Ultrasound scan of an infant hip. Baseline drawn along the ilium (1), bony acetabulum (2), cartilaginous labrum (3). The α angle formed measures the bony acetabulum. The β angle assesses the cartilaginous angle. Both angles are normal in this example. The dotted circle outlines the cartilaginous femoral head. Approximately half the femoral head should be 'below' line 1 and covered by the bony acetabulum. (b) Ultrasound scan of a dysplastic infant hip pretreatment with a Pavlik harness. The α angle is 53°. (c) Ultrasound scan of an infant hip after treatment with a Pavlik harness. The α angle is now 60°.

Interpretation of the radiographs may be difficult in this age group but there are several features that should be noted (**Figure 2.4**).

Hilgenreiner's line is drawn through the triradiate cartilage of both hips and sets the horizontal axis. Perkin's lines are at 90° to this axis and are drawn in line with the lateral most extent of the visible bony acetabulum. These lines divide each hip radiographically into quadrants and the femoral head should lie in the inferomedial quadrant.

Shenton's line should be seen as a smooth curve going around the obturator foramen with a seamless transition to follow the curve of the medial femoral neck.

The acetabular index (the inclination of the line drawn along the ossified bony acetabular roof relative to Hilgenreiner's line) is another important measurement in children's hips (**Figure 2.4**). Its value decreases as ossification continues and the hip grows older. It is used to monitor the response of the hip to treatment. Debate continues about what angles constitute normal reflecting the appreciation of DDH as a spectrum. Tonnis set some age-related standards [15]; values between 1–2 standard deviations indicate a delay in ossification, and values greater than this signify dysplasia [16].

Other radiographic measures are used in the adolescent after ossification of the triradiate cartilage.

Serial radiographs along with clinical examination form the cornerstone of our Stanmore surveillance protocol as described in the literature [17]. There is a balance to be struck between regular surveillance and limiting radiation exposure with one study suggesting a small but slightly increased risk of leukaemias in patients treated with surgery for DDH, whom they presume to have been exposed to serial radiographs [18].

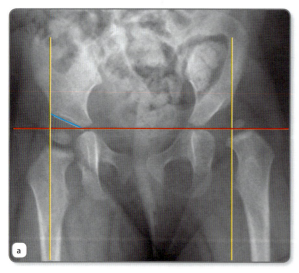 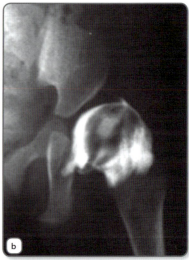

Figure 2.4 (a) Radiographic assessment of developmental dysplasia of the hips (DDH) on an anteroposterior pelvic radiograph. Hilgenreiner's line (red) passes through the open triradiate cartilages of both hips to mark the horizontal, Perkin's line (yellow) is perpendicular and vertical at the edge of the depicted bony acetabulum. The acetabular index is the inclination of the line drawn along the ossified bony acetabular roof (blue on the normal side) relative to Hilgenreiner's line. The ossific nucleus should be located in the inferior medial quadrant formed by the intersection of Hilgenreiner's and Perkin's lines. In this example, the ossific nucleus of the left hip is outside this quadrant and the nucleus is smaller in size: both signs of DDH. (b) A hip arthrogram more accurately demonstrates the cartilaginous acetabulum and femoral head and permits a dynamic assessment under anaesthesia. The white area represents dye between the subluxed femoral head and the acetabulum.

TREATMENT

The principal aim of early treatment for DDH is to achieve a concentric reduction of the hip and facilitate stable movement while avoiding complications. The hip has a tremendous ability to remodel and 'normalise' if provided with optimum conditions, especially if those conditions can be provided early in infancy and we know that many cases of neonatal instability and dysplasia resolve spontaneously without treatment.

There is surprisingly little evidence to say that early treatment is more effective than the natural history of hip instability, but those treated before 7 weeks fare better than those treated later.

Outcomes decline the later the diagnosis is made, perhaps due to the greater need for more extensive treatments with greater risks and complications.

With respect to DDH, the spectrum of severity, stability and anatomical differences on both the acetabular and femoral sides, combined with differing responses to similar treatments, makes it difficult to outline a robust prescriptive treatment protocol. Instead, the following sections outline the treatment principles used at various stages of the pathophysiology.

Pavlik harness and splinting

In accordance with our principal aim for treatment stated above, infant hips deemed to require treatment to obtain and maintain the reduction of the femoral head within the acetabulum (Ortolani positive hips) or to improve stability (Barlow positive hips) may be treated with a harness or splint. Rigid splints such as the Von Rosen have been shown to be successful but the most popular treatment is dynamic splinting with the Pavlik harness (**Figure 2.5**).

In the presence of hip dislocation or instability, treatment usually commences between 2 and 3 weeks although some specialist centres will wait until 6 weeks: treatment of a neonatally detected hip instability should not be delayed past this point (without the agreement of your treating team).

The Pavlik harness is a dynamic, flexion/abduction orthosis that is fully adjustable both to suit the size of the patient and to accommodate the best position for his/her particular hip morphology.

Great care must be taken when using this method of treatment for an Ortolani negative hip (the irreducible dislocation): some centres would not use a harness for such a case and many would treat for only 1–2 weeks if no progress was seen.

For the Ortolani positive and Barlow positive hips, the hip is placed in the reduced position and held in the middle of the safe/stable zone of flexion/extension, abduction/adduction. The arc of movement is 'controlled' by the anterior and posterior harness straps. Extreme positions and excessive forces must be avoided as they risk compromising the vascularity of the femoral head. Avascular necrosis can be a devastating problem in the infant hip causing a stiff and painful hip from childhood onwards. The risk of avascular necrosis has been reported as low as 0.3% [19] and is minimised by careful and considered application and use of the splint.

The harness encourages a gradual stretch of the tight adductor muscles and with increasing abduction, relocation of the femoral head is more likely and the Ortolani negative hip may become an Ortolani positive hip; similarly the Ortolani positive hip may become a Barlow positive hip. The reduction can be gradual and by permitting movement,

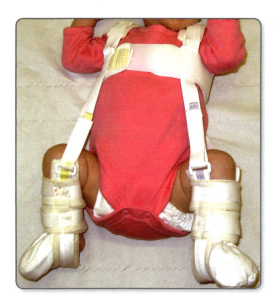

Figure 2.5 Baby in Pavlik harness.

growth of the acetabulum is promoted and the socket deepens to accept the femoral head. Once the hip is reduced, it is maintained until joint stability and normal (near-normal) anatomy are achieved. The stretched and lax joint capsule 'shrinks' and muscle length and tone improve.

In our institution, the harness is applied between the ages of 2 and 6 weeks for a period of 6–8 weeks, but protocols vary considerably and there is no single best practice method. The success rates quoted may be as high as 95% of cases but this will vary with the case mix treated: the treatment of the Ortolani positive and negative hips is often less successful than treatment of the Barlow positive hips.

In many centres, treatment protocols are driven more by the Graf classification than the clinical interpretation of the pathology.

The success of the splint diminishes and is questionable between 4 and 6 months of age and generally not appropriate after 6 months of age. It is also contraindicated in hips which are teratologic and not reducible, or in whom there is poor compliance.

The splint is worn 23–24 hours per day during the treatment period and the response is assessed on ultrasound at 2–3 weekly intervals. Failure of reduction after 2–3 weeks in the splint is an indication to discontinue splinting. The baby must also be assessed clinically to adjust the splint for growth and to ensure there is no femoral nerve palsy (**Figure 2.5**) [20].

Closed reduction

For those diagnosed late or those in whom early treatment has been unsuccessful, a closed reduction under general anaesthetic forms the next level in the treatment ladder. This is often coupled with an arthrogram which outlines the cartilaginous parts of the joint and allows a radiographic dynamic assessment of the hip to be performed, and the soft tissue 'blocks' to obtaining and maintaining a reduction can be evaluated (**Table 2.4**).

If the hip reduces, surgical release of adductor longus and psoas may improve the quality of the reduction and its stability. The reduction is then held by placing the child in a hip spica cast (**Figure 2.6**). Both legs have to be included in the cast and the plaster may end at the knee or at the ankle.

Table 2.4 Structures obstructing reduction	
Site of obstruction	**Obstructing tissue**
Extracapsular	Adductor muscles
	Psoas muscle
Capsule	Hourglass constriction which prevents the femoral head relocating
Intracapsular	Ligamentum teres
	Transverse acetabular ligament
	Pulvinar and infolded labrum

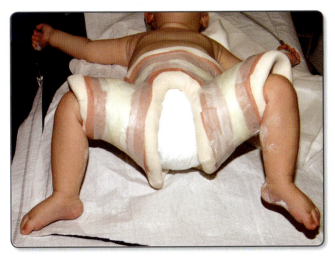

Figure 2.6 A short leg hip cast.

Table 2.5 Factors affecting joint stability	
Factors	**Characteristics**
Bony anatomy	Are the femoral head and acetabulum well matched in terms of shape, size and orientation?
Soft tissue integrity	Are the stabilising ligaments and capsule working well?
Muscle tone	Are the muscles long enough and working well enough?

Following the procedure, maintenance of the reduction is with imaging; debate continues as to whether plain radiographs, limited slice computed tomography, magnetic resonance imaging or USS provide the most appropriate information.

Joint stability depends on three factors: bony anatomy, soft tissue integrity and muscle tone (**Table 2.5**).

The duration of cast treatment varies from centre to centre: it does take time for the stretched capsule to shrink and to provide stability for the joint and for the acetabulum and femoral head/neck to remodel to a perfect shape. Our protocol is for 12 weeks in plaster cast followed by 6 weeks in a removable brace. Some surgeons advocate much longer in plaster but there is little robust evidence for this. The use of traction preoperatively has fallen out of favour in the United Kingdom but it is still popular in Europe.

Open reduction

The inability to obtain or maintain a closed reduction of a hip is an indication for an open reduction. Age and the surgeon's understanding of the individual pathophysiology may also be indications for open surgery.

Open reduction of the hip may be performed via a medial (groin) incision and approach or via an anterior (bikini-cut) incision below the iliac crest. The appropriate approach is chosen depending on which soft tissue blocks need to be dealt with and whether or not the surgeon wishes to take the opportunity to surgically 'shrink' the capsule and/or change the shape of the bones to improve the hip joint stability.

Following the open reduction, a hip spica cast is applied extending to the ankle on the affected side; the total time in cast varies from 6 to 10 weeks.

Late presentation

The older the child is at presentation and the longer the hip has been out of joint, the greater the likelihood that more extensive surgery will be required to obtain and maintain the hip in the reduced position. Realignment of the acetabulum and the femoral head by means of a pelvic and/or femoral osteotomy is common when the child is aged 2 years or more (**Figure 2.7**).

A femoral osteotomy results in a change in the rotational profile of the bone; as a result of this, the child may have less internal rotation ability postoperatively and may, e.g. no longer be able to 'W-sit'.

A pelvic osteotomy reorientates or reshapes the acetabulum so that it faces the correct way and is the correct size; various eponymous names are given to these operations. As a very general rule, the more surgery that is required to reduce the hip, the poorer the long term outcome is likely to be.

Ongoing evaluation

Once a hip is relocated, it is the hope of every surgeon that the child's growth potential and innate 'understanding' of how a hip should be will aid in hip development; this

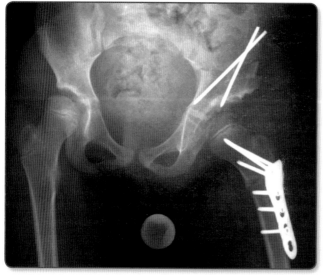

Figure 2.7 Anteroposterior pelvic radiograph showing a left hip that has been treated for developmental dysplasia of the hips with an open reduction and pelvic and femoral osteotomies.

may not always take place and thus regular follow-up until skeletal maturity may be required.

Even in the presence of a normally functioning, asymptomatic child, further surgery may be indicated to correct, e.g. residual dysplasia or a persisting leg length difference or to alter the natural history of any growth disturbances caused by the surgery. Avascular necrosis and infection remain the most feared complications of surgery for DDH.

SCREENING AND THE FUTURE

The debate about screening for DDH continues. It has been acknowledged that neither the clinical nor ultrasound screening programmes, currently in use, fulfil the World Health Organization criteria for a successful screening programme. Thus, we should be discussing surveillance programmes for DDH rather than screening programmes.

In the United Kingdom, the 1986 Standing Medical Advisory Committee recommendations have been recently superseded by the implementation of the NHS (National Health Service) Newborn and Infant Physical Examination Programme (NIPE) in 2008 which incorporates a requirement for training personnel and appraising the effectiveness of the programme. The NIPE recommends that the hips are checked clinically within the first 72 hours of life and between 6 and 8 weeks of age; the only risk factors mandating an USS were breech presentation and a strong family history.

A Medical Research Council study demonstrated that 93% of trusts in this country screen clinically with selective ultrasound assessment of those infants at high risk. The definition of high risk varies from centre to centre as does the percentage of the newborn population who are screened [21]. In contrast, in Coventry, universal USS takes place. On average, 98% of babies are scanned within 48 hours of birth; although 6% had abnormalities requiring a review at 6 weeks, their overall treatment rate was lower than many selective screening programmes. There have been no known late diagnoses in this cohort of patients [22].

Universal USS often leads to a higher rate of splint treatment along with a presumed increase in complications such avascular necrosis and femoral nerve palsy. Nevertheless, as shown in both Germany and Austria, the adoption of such a policy has resulted in a reduction in the number of children requiring surgery for DDH [23].

There have been two randomised controlled trials comparing selective versus universal US screening [24,25]. Although both failed to demonstrate a significant difference, there was a trend towards more late cases in the selective groups. In both studies, the clinical examination was performed by trained and experienced clinicians, and it has been shown in several studies that clinical screening programmes are more effective when the examiner is experienced [25]. While there are no studies commenting on the effectiveness of USS programmes in relation to the experience of the sonographers, it is likely that the same conclusions could be drawn.

In the United Kingdom, there is evidence from several studies that contemporary screening/surveillance programmes are not being implemented well. Those presenting late may have been failed by the existing programmes and are thus more likely to need extensive treatment. It is also true that those presenting late often do not have the risk factors of breech or a family history, as such cases have already been screened. Thus, it is the absence of risk factors that is in itself a risk factor when assessing a child over the age of 3–4 months. The 2012 study by Sanghrajka et al confirmed that 71% of those who came to surgical treatment of their DDH had presented late [26]. A large number of patients in both groups were female and first born. Perhaps, female gender does need to be considered a risk factor. This could effectively restrict universal USS programmes to the 50% of the population who are at most risk and those who are at high risk from their history and examination. It is important to consider the USS as an investigation which addresses the question, is this hip normal? In this context, it is clear that the value of an investigation is only appreciated when it is combined with the history and physical examination.

As a profession and as a society, it is important that we decide on the most effective and efficient way in managing our patients with DDH. DDH may not be a preventable condition, but it is a detectable condition and early treatment is more effective than late treatment. Our clinical detection rates must improve, and while universal US surveillance programmes may be expensive so are the costs of delayed diagnosis, not only in terms of physical and mental scars but also the financial implications of repeated surgical procedures and medicolegal claims.

Key points for clinical practice

- DDH represents a continuum of hip pathology ranging from mild dysplasia to frank dislocations that may be irreducible.
- Many mildly dysplastic hips with or without instability will go on to stabilise and develop normally without intervention.
- Clinical examination is critical and should be performed by a smaller number of experienced clinicians, be they paediatricians, orthopaedic surgeons, specialist physiotherapists or specialist nurses who are well versed in the diagnosis and treatment of DDH.
- Early diagnosis and intervention before the age of 6 weeks frequently involves harness treatment for 6 weeks with low failure rates and few complications.
- Late diagnosis is often associated with multiple surgical procedures and, ultimately, a less favourable outcome.
- DDH is a factor in 30% of total hip arthroplasties performed in patients under 60 years.
- Contemporary UK surveillance programmes for DDH require improvements in design and implementation.

REFERENCES

1.   Klisic P. Congenital dislocation of the hip – a misleading term. J Bone Joint Surg Br 1989; 71B:136.
2.   Dezateux C, Rosendahl K. Developmental dysplasia of the hip. Lancet 2007; 369: 1541–1552.
3.   Andersson J, Vogel I, Uldbjerg N. Serum 17 beta-estradiol in newborn and neonatal hip instability. J Pediatr Orthop 2002; 22:88–91.
4.   Blatt SH. Joined at the hip? A paleoepidemiological study of developmental dysplasia of the hip and its relation to swaddling practices among indigenous peoples of North America. Am J Hum Biol 2013; 25:821–834.
5.   Kramer AA, Berg K, Nance WE. Familial aggregation of congenital dislocation of the hip in a Norwegian population. J Clin Epidemiol 1988; 41:91–96.
6.   Smith D, Aase J. Polygenic inheritance of certain common malformations. Evidence and empiric recurrence risk data. J Paediatr 1970; 76:653–659.
7.   Yamamuro T, Ishida K. Recent advances in the prevention, early diagnosis, and treatment of congenital dislocation of the hip in Japan. Clin Orthop Relat Res 1984; 184:34–40.
8.   Wald N, Leck I. Antenatal and neonatal Screening, 2nd edition. Oxford: Oxford University Press, 2000.
9.   Holroyd B, Wedge J. Developmental dysplasia of the hip. Orthop Trauma 2009; 23:162–168.
10. Clark NMP. The diagnosis and management of congenital dislocation of the hip. Curr Orthop 2004; 18:256 –261.

11. Barlow TG. Early diagnosis and treatment of congenital dislocation of the hip. J Bone Jt Surg Br 1962;44-B:292–301.
12. Jones D. An assessment of the value of examination of the hip in the newborn. J Bone Joint Surg Br 1977; 59:318–322.
13. Choudry Q, Goyal R, Paton RW. Is limitation of hip abduction a useful clinical sign in the diagnosis of developmental dysplasia of the hip? Arch Dis Child 2013; 98:862–866.
14. Clarke NM, Harcke HT, McHugh P, et al. Real-time ultrasound in the diagnosis of congenital dislocation and dysplasia of the hip. J Bone Joint Surg Br 1985; 67:406–412.
15. Tönnis D, Brunken D. Differentiation of normal and pathological acetabular roof angle in the diagnosis of hip dysplasia. Evaluation of 2294 acetabular roof angles of hip joints in children. Arch Orthop Unfallchir 1968; 64:197–228.
16. United Kingdom National Screening Committee (NSC). Child Health Sub-Group Report: dysplasia of the hip, September. 2004. London; NSC, 2004.
17. Wright J, Tudor F, Luff T, et al. Surveillance after treatment of children with developmental dysplasia of the hip: current UK practice and the proposed Stanmore protocol. J Pediatr Orthop B 2013; 22:509–515.
18. Bone C, Hsieh G. The risk of carcinogenesis from raadiographs to pediatric orthopaedic patients. J Pediatr Orthop 2000; 20:251–254.
19. Taylor GR, Clarke NM. Monitoring the treatment of developmental dysplasia of the hip with the Pavlik harness. The role of ultrasound. J Bone Joint Surg Br 1997; 79:719–723.
20. Viere RG, Birch JG, Herring JA, et al. Use of the Pavlik harness in congenital dislocation of the hip. An analysis of failures of treatment. J Bone Joint Surg Am 1990; 72:238–244.
21. Eastwood DM. Neonatal hip screening. Lancet 2003; 361:595–597.
22. Marks DS, Clegg J, al-Chalabi AN. Routine ultrasound screening for neonatal hip instability. Can it abolish late-presenting congenital dislocation of the hip? J Bone Joint Surg Br 1994; 76:534–538.
23. Ihme N, Altenhofen L, von Kries R, et al. [Hip ultrasound screening in Germany. Results and comparison with other screening procedures]. Orthopade 2008; 37:541–546, 548–549.
24. Rosendahl K, Markestad T, Lie RT. Ultrasound screening for developmental dysplasia of the hip in the neonate: the effect on treatment rate and prevalence of late cases. Pediatrics 1994; 94:47–52.
25. Holen KJ, Tegnander A, Bredland T, et al. Universal or selective screening of the neonatal hip using ultrasound? A prospective, randomised trial of 15,529 newborn infants. J Bone Joint Surg Br 2002; 84:886–90.
26. Sanghrajka AP, Murnaghan CF, Shekkeris A, et al. Open reduction for developmental dysplasia of the hip: failures of screening or failures of treatment? Ann R Coll Surg Engl 2013; 95:113–117.

Chapter 3

Sport and exercise medicine for health in children

Bhavesh D Kumar, Charlotte Hamlyn Williams, Julian Redhead

INTRODUCTION

The specialty of sport and exercise medicine (SEM) centres on the promotion and facilitation of safe sport, exercise and physical activity (PA) for improved health and well-being. This includes diagnosis, management and prevention of injuries and illness related to exercise, and the promotion and prescription of PA. This chapter explores the benefits of PA in children and reviews important medical and musculoskeletal conditions related to childhood exercise.

SEM is a developing field for all clinicians owing to the significant benefits that PA and exercise can have on children's health.

Though the terms are often used interchangeably, exercise refers to any planned, structured repetitive body movement undertaken to improve physical fitness, and PA refers to any body movement produced by skeletal muscles that requires energy expenditure.

In the UK, evidence-based Department of Health guidelines recommend that children and youth aged 5–17 should accumulate at least 60 minutes of moderate to vigorous PA daily, with additional time providing greater health benefits. More vigorous intensity activities that strengthen muscle and bone should be incorporated at least three times per week.

BENEFITS OF BEING PHYSICALLY ACTIVE

Regular moderate intensity PA for children, such as walking, cycling or participating in sports, has significant benefits for health. These include the development of healthy musculoskeletal tissues and cardiovascular system, maintenance of healthy weight, and reducing immediate- and long-term risk of noncommunicable diseases, including cardiovascular disease (CVD), cancer and diabetes.

Psychological benefits include enhanced self-esteem, self-confidence and self-efficacy, as well as helping improve social skills, extending social networks and reducing anxiety and the potential for reducing depression.

Bhavesh D Kumar MRCS MRCGP FFSEM Institute of Sport Exercise and Health, University College London, London, UK

Charlotte Hamlyn Williams PhD, Institute of Child Health, University College London, London, UK

Julian Redhead FRCP FCEM MFSEM, Emergency Department, St Mary's Hospital, London, UK. Email: julian.redhead@imperial.nhs.uk (for correspondence)

PHYSICAL INACTIVITY

Current evidence suggests that children and young people in the developed world are not participating in enough PA [1] and are missing out on the benefits. Health surveys in England have revealed that only 32% of boys and 24% of girls aged 2–15 living in England meet recommended guidelines [2] and an average of one third of children aged 10 and 11 are overweight or obese. Physical inactivity (PIA) has been identified as the fourth leading risk factor for global mortality causing an estimated 3.2 million deaths globally [3] and increasing UK National Health Service (NHS) spending by £1.48 billion per year [4]. Impact from reduced quality of life and life expectancy is estimated to cost £10,000 per child [5].

The effects of exercise on cardiovascular risk factors in children have yet to be studied as extensively as within the adult population. There is, however, mounting evidence suggesting that increasing PA, particularly from no activity to even a little regular activity, provides the greatest health gains (**Figure 3.1**) [6], improving blood pressure, lipid profile, insulin sensitivity and endothelial function. It is thus critical to engage children in PA as part of their everyday life at a time when long-term behaviour patterns are developing.

SEDENTARY BEHAVIOUR

The amount of time spent in very low energy expenditure states during awake hours, such as sitting or lying down, is now considered a health risk factor independent of time spent undertaking PA. Studies show that 2-hour daily television viewing is associated with a 20% increased risk of type 2 diabetes and 13% increased risk of all-cause mortality in adulthood [7]. Compared with those reporting <4 hours of total daily sitting time, those who spend 10 or more hours per day seated have a significantly greater body mass index, waist circumference, systolic and diastolic blood pressure, serum cholesterol and triglycerides and nonfasting blood sugar [8]. Such findings have led to guidance advocating minimising sedentary time for extended periods from childhood.

PHYSICAL ACTIVITY IN CHILDREN WITH LONG-TERM CONDITIONS

The problem of PIA is further intensified for the 10–15% of children living with long-term conditions (LTCs), who on the whole fall short of minimum recommended levels

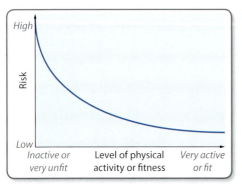

Figure 3.1 Dose–response relationship between the amount of physical activity and health benefits accrued. Adapted from Department of Health [6].

of PA. Despite the challenges and additional barriers that may exist, these children can experience many of the same health benefits as their healthy peers. In conditions such as type 1 diabetes or asthma, PA is an essential component of their overall treatment plan [9]. Many of the comorbidities associated with LTC including obesity, respiratory infections, depression, poor bone health, eating disorders, psychological disorders and an increased risk of CVD could be managed or improved through increasing PA [9-11].

IS EXERCISE SAFE FOR CHILDREN WITH LONG-TERM CONDITIONS?

Some health professionals are cautious about prescribing exercise to children and young people with LTC because of concerns over the risks involved. These range from seizure induction in children with epilepsy and breathlessness in asthma or cystic fibrosis, to hypoglycaemia or ketoacidosis in insulin-dependent diabetes and dehydration in chronic renal failure. In reality, for the overwhelming majority of patients, in which the medical condition is well managed, the patients and parents have a good understanding of the condition, and abrupt escalations in PA are avoided with proper warm-up and cool down; exercise is very safe, with the benefits far outweighing the potential risks.

The rate of exercise-associated collapse or death in children is exceedingly low. The incidence of sudden cardiac death in children aged 12–19 playing sport is an estimated 1.45 and 0.66 per 100,000 athletes per year in boys and girls respectively [12]. Risks are highest in those who have been chronically sedentary and undertake vigorous exercise abruptly and those with symptoms of or confirmed cardiovascular conditions. Ethnicity-related differences may exist.

A physician-led participation physical evaluation (PPE) is advisable for all children with known LTC. This comprises an up-to-date history (including a probing personal history of cardiac-related symptoms and a family history of unexplained collapse or death before the age of 35) and physical examination (including general medical, cardiovascular and musculoskeletal). The purpose is to identify those who need further diagnostic tests, counselling or rehabilitation.

Apparently healthy but thus far inactive children can be screened more simply with the help of a short children's PA readiness questionnaire, to help identify risk factors that may require a PPE via the appropriate specialist, sports physician or sports cardiologist. They can arrange further tests and risk stratification to facilitate appropriate counselling as to the types of activities, level of supervision and medical facilities recommended to facilitate safer exercise.

There are a small number of conditions in which certain types or intensities of exercise, and rarely all exercise, are contraindicated by expert consensus [13]. These include uncontrolled cardiac, metabolic, inflammatory or infectious disease, in which the risks of PA are deemed disproportionately high. Once controlled, exercise may form an effective part of their rehabilitation.

EXERCISE TESTING

Physical fitness and aerobic capacity is an important determinant of overall health. Exercise testing can provide a valuable, noninvasive tool to evaluate physical fitness throughout childhood and adolescence [14]. For example, group testing can be conducted in schools (e.g. a 20 m shuttle run or a bleep test) with results used to monitor progress as well as screen and identify children that may be struggling for whom a medical assessment and further exercise testing may be warranted. A growing number of sports medicine and anaesthetic departments have provisions for laboratory-based exercise testing using a modified Bruce protocol treadmill test or cardiopulmonary exercise test with expired gas analysis. This can help determine the level of functional impairment to the cardiovascular, respiratory or metabolic systems, and help quantify appropriate training zones or activity intensity that would be deemed safe and effective.

CARDIAC SCREENING

This aims to uncover significant structural or conduction-related abnormalities that are relatively infrequent in the population, but can increase the risk of sudden death. A dozen or so young people die suddenly each week in the United Kingdom of previously undetected heart problems. Though most do not occur during exercise, PA, particularly at vigorous intensities, is known to transiently increase the risk of collapse or death in those who are susceptible. Patients, who are symptomatic of a possible cardiac condition, and those who have had a family member died suddenly under the age of 35 are eligible for NHS screening by referral to a cardiologist, preferably one with a sports cardiology interest. Screening generally includes a thorough history, cardiovascular examination and echocardiography (ECG). ECG, exercise testing and other special tests may be indicated in some. Risk stratification for exercise and appropriate counselling are key outcomes.

There is considerable controversy over whether to screen patients who lie outside of these criteria, from what age and how extensively. Factors debated include the relatively low prevalence of abnormalities, cost, and false positive and false negative detection rates, which can have implications for sports participation, mortgage and life insurance applications. Those participating in elite sport are often offered cardiac screening on one or more occasions after the age of 14 via the sport's governing bodies or professional clubs.

PRESCRIBING EXERCISE

Exercise is vital medicine. The Department of Health (England) [15] and Chief Medical Officer [16] stress the importance of PA for children's health and highlight that efforts need to be made to increase participation in PA and promote evidence-based innovative solutions to overcome PIA and SB. PA patterns in childhood track into adulthood [17] highlighting the need to promote and facilitate beneficial PA behaviours as early as possible.

Engaging the child in a discussion about PA in a skilled manner is key in helping improve the patient health and quality of life and in many cases the trajectory of chronic disease.

Every child should be asked about PA and SB as part of the social history, and documented in daily or weekly time and intensity units.

PA intensity is divided into light, moderate, vigorous or very vigorous. These can be classified scientifically on the basis of formal exercise testing, but for practical purposes, light exercise corresponds to standing or strolling intensities, and moderate intensity (e.g. brisk walking, gentle cycling or roller blading) can be distinguished from vigorous (e.g. running or shovelling) by the sing–talk test. During moderate-intensity exercise, a person should be able to talk in sentences but not sing; at vigorous intensities, neither is possible. Competitive sport usually entails very vigorous intensities of PA. Moderate- and vigorous-intensity PA (MVPA) is recommended as being most beneficial to health, though there is increasing evidence for the considerable beneficial effects of light activities in comparison to sedentary time.

The following points are tips for increasing health, and promoting physical activity for children outside of school:

- Encourage parents to leave 10–20 minutes earlier for the school run, and walk part of the way, helping build social links and motivating factors
- Engender a sense of achievement, by praising new competences in sport or good performance
- Competitive sport facilitates enjoyment and participation from early adolescence
- Promote family exercise, e.g. dog walking or cycling
- Use local parks or green spaces where children can make new friends
- Signpost to web-based PA information hubs, such as the local council or British Heart Foundation
- Technology within smartphones, watches and tablets can encourage and monitor PA levels and biometric data
- Engage local authorities involved in supporting and planning an active environment such as cycle lanes and green spaces
  For exercise prescription, the following tips are useful:
- Ask at each consultation how many minutes of MVPA a child is currently undertaking daily. Many now consider this measure an essential vital sign
- For those who do not undertake any regular PA, use a short PA readiness questionnaire, with parental help if necessary
- Stable and well-managed conditions should have no contraindications for exercise
- Children with new LTC diagnoses can benefit from direct medical supervision and guidance when commencing exercise, e.g. in a clinical exercise facility or laboratory. This can help instil confidence with exercise for the child and parents, allowing them to become familiar with normal cardiorespiratory responses to exercise and the precautions and preparations that might be necessary
- Identify solutions to circumnavigate nonmedical barriers to taking up or increasing PA
- The type of activity advised should be based on what the children enjoy, their capabilities, their motivations, availability of equipment or facilities, their daily routine and family or social environment
- Initially encourage PA of moderate intensity in bouts of at least 10 minutes in which they should be able to talk and be active at the same time
- Gradual progression should be encouraged, in terms of frequency, intensity, time and type (FITT) of activity. Once the child is comfortable with PA at a certain level and his/her LTC is stable, increase one of the four components of FITT each week
- Always commence exercise with a warm-up, allowing the cardiorespiratory system to respond gradually, reducing any small risk of injury or adverse cardiac event. Equally, reduce activity level slowly at the end of a session
- Break up periods of 30 minutes of continuous sitting time during homework or screen time by a 1-minute stand and stretch or visit to another room

SPECIFIC INJURIES IN CHILDHOOD

Head injuries

These injuries are relatively common during participation in sports and other recreational activities. Concussion is a prevalent subset of head injury characterised by transiently impaired neurological function rather than structural injury. It can resolve quickly and spontaneously in the majority of cases, particularly, if recognised and managed appropriately with complete physical and cognitive rest until symptoms resolve. This might require time away from academic activities (this is an active area of research). Loss of consciousness need not be a feature, and symptoms can include a change to the child's normal cognitive or emotional state or sleep pattern. The Sport Concussion Assessment Tool version 3 (SCAT 3) is a useful tool to help clinicians diagnose and manage suspected concussion. The Child-SCAT 3 is tailored for children aged 5-12.

Concussion can result from a significant biomechanical force to any part of the body transmitting a force to the brain. Estimates of incidence are limited by the relatively loose definition of concussion and challenges with recognition and reporting. Horse riding, rugby and soccer have relatively high incidences. It has been suggested that the increased head-to-neck ratio and weaker cervical musculature puts a child's brain at a greater risk of injury than an adult for the same impact force.

Children take longer to recover from concussion than adults and complications such as malignant cerebral oedema only occur in the paediatric population [18]. It is also hypothesised that the developing brain with decreased myelination is more susceptible to longer term sequelae. In postconcussion syndrome, e.g. symptoms may persist for over a month, postulated to result from altered neurotransmitter function. Imaging is indicated via referral to a neurologist or sports physician to exclude gross trauma when patients fail to show improvement. In the absence of specific guidelines, persistent symptoms beyond 10 days seem a sensible time to consider referral. There is increasing evidence of the long-term consequences from single, and perhaps more importantly, multiple concussion episodes. The younger the child is exposed to potential head injuries, the more likely the recurrent concussion episodes will occur.

Traditionally, advice regarding head injuries has confined itself to the acute deterioration of the child, e.g. with increasing headache, vomiting or fluctuating consciousness. Doctors who are likely to treat children following head injuries should expand head injury advice to 'return to sport' guidance [19,20]. Children should expect to go through a gradual, stepwise approach to return to play, as outlined in **Table 3.1**.

Table 3.1 Graduated return to play following concussion	
Stage	**Activity level**
1	No activity
2	Light aerobic activity, e.g. walking
3	Heavier aerobic activity, e.g. running
4	Noncontact sport specific drills
5	Contact sport specific drills
6	Return to full participation

Children must be symptom free as they move from one stage to the next, no faster than every 24 hours. Although there is no evidence base for how long this should take, most doctors involved in sports allow 6–10 days from when initial symptoms resolve [21]. Recurrence of symptoms at any stage mandates immediate physical and cognitive rest for at least 24 hours, before a trial of return to the last stage at which the child was asymptomatic.

It is important to note that self-reported symptoms may not correspond to full resolution of symptoms when assessed by neurocognitive testing. In organised sport, there is a move to baseline neurocognitive testing for all participants to help with decisions regarding return to play.

Protection of children from head injuries should also be considered. Children grow by a series of growth spurts, with maximum growth acceleration during puberty. There can be a significant mismatch in size between children of the same age group, which can contribute to injury risk particularly in contact sports. Thus competitive contact sports should consider the size and development of the participants rather than their age. The use of protective equipment to protect against potential head injuries should also be encouraged in some sports [21].

Acute avulsion injuries

Growth spurts are also recognised as a time of increased risk of injury for other reasons [22]. The increasing length of limbs often results in a child who is less balanced and coordinated. Bone lengthening occurs before the muscle tendon unit; the muscle increases in strength before the tendon; greater forces act on the moving limb due to the poor coordination; the process of endochondral ossification leaves the tendon–bone junction susceptible to injury. All these factors result in the bone being weaker than the muscle and tendon connecting them, resulting in a propensity for avulsion injuries rather than muscle injuries in children.

The most common avulsion injuries are related to the larger muscles; the hamstring attachment to the ischeal tuberosity, the rectus femoris muscle attachment to the anterior inferior iliac spine or the sartorius muscle attachment to the anterior superior iliac spine. Though, there is also evidence of the benefits of exercise on bone maturity, which can be advantageous in reducing injury risk in later life [23].

The child will usually present with a sudden episode of pain and disability. The pain is often felt along the tendon, although the main area of tenderness will usually be related to the avulsion site. A plain X-ray may identify the bony fragment if large enough. Computed tomography (CT) scanning is avoided where possible owing to high-radiation doses. Magnetic resonance imaging (MRI) can usually identify most subtle soft tissue injuries and fractures.

In general, avulsion fractures are treated conservatively with the child resuming activities as pain allows. An important exception is the attachment of the anterior cruciate ligament to the tibial spine. This may require surgical reduction and needs to be actively investigated if suspected.

Avulsion injuries are being increasingly recognised as intensity of training increases and some sports become increasingly professionalised [24]. There are concerns that intensive periods of training can have long-term effects on the developing child, although recent evidence suggests that resistance training is safe and effective especially following puberty [25]. However training programmes should take into account the growth pattern of the individual child, the need for appropriate recovery time and nutrition to fuel both growth and exercise without comprising either.

Susceptibility to injury can also be lessened through injury-prevention exercise programmes focussing on common sites of injury within the chosen sport, addressing factors including strength, balance, coordination, flexibility and agility [26]. The highest level of evidence for effectiveness exists among team ball sports, though achieving adequate compliance appears one of the greatest challenges yet to be overcome.

OSTEOCHONDROSIS

The term osteochondrosis refers to a collection of disorders where there is derangement of the normal growth of the epiphyses [27]. They occur exclusively in children, except for osteochondritis dissecans, which can occur in adults and does not truly involve the growth centre. Previous classification of these conditions has involved the possible pathological cause of the injury (e.g. traction apophysitis); however, more recent classifications have used the site of injury. Many have an eponym (**Table 3.2**).

Diagnosis is usually clinical and supported by radiography where doubt exists. The conditions are often related to increased intensity of training. Almost all will resolve over time with appropriate rest and modified training load; however, they account for a significant time loss from both training and competition, and can adversely affect the long-term ambitions of the young athlete.

One of the most common examples is Osgood–Schlatter disease, occurring early in adolescence. The pathogenesis of this condition remains unclear. Recent papers have described the presence of neovessels being associated with more severe disease, perhaps due to the association of nerve fibres with the vessels [28]. The patient will describe general knee pain during activity, although tenderness is usually isolated to the tibial tuberosity at the insertion of the patella tendon. Treatment programmes have traditionally involved immobilisation and rest of the affected joint, with some success.

However, such a period of inactivity results in loss of fitness, disruption to sports development, and may accrue towards negative cardiometabolic health consequences. More recent approaches have involved continued participation in exercise with a scoring system according to pain. When the pain is severe, complete rest would be advisable. Modified training can continue with relative protection of the affected area if the pain is moderate, and mild pain can allow full participation according to tolerance. Taping techniques and muscle-strengthening programmes have been found to benefit some patients.

BACK PAIN IN ATHLETIC CHILDREN

Studies in both the USA and Europe have identified nonspecific low back pain in children with rising prevalence. There is evidence that the symptoms can become recurrent and

Table 3.2 Examples of osteochondroses	
Eponym	Location
Perthes	Femoral head
Osgood–Schlatter	Tibial tuberosity
Blount's	Proximal tibia

debilitating. Weakness of the lumbo-pelvic and abdominal core muscles and poor spinal mobility has been associated with episodes of low back pain [29]. Specific exercise can improve neuromuscular control in these areas as part of the treatment and prevention of low back pain in adolescents.

Stress fractures are being increasingly recognised in children participating in sports, with higher incidences in gymnastics, cricket and rugby. A stress fracture of the pars interarticularis (spondylolysis) involving the lamina of the spinal vertebra is important to recognise. Spondylolysis incidence of 4.4–5.2% in children has been documented with increased rates being observed in athletic adolescents [30]. The concern with unrecognised and untreated spondylolysis is progression to spondylolisthesis, characterised by forward displacement of one vertebral body on another.

Spondylolysis is usually associated with extension and rotational stresses, and clinical examination will usually demonstrate exacerbation of the pain when repeating these forces on the child's back in a controlled manner. Pathology can be confirmed with plain radiographs, though, in most cases, the initial investigation is now an MRI, due to the greater sensitivity, absence of radiation and the potential to identify other pathology. Negative findings out of keeping with clinical suspicion may necessitate CT or single-photon emission CT scan which can help identify active lesions. Studies have confirmed that many lesions detected on imaging are asymptomatic.

The majority of lesions occur in the fourth or fifth lumbar vertebrae. Most patients have good outcomes with conservative treatment including rest, core muscle training and progressive rehabilitation for return to sport. However, there is no consensus or well-designed trials on their overall management. It is accepted that evidence of bone healing is not necessary for the patient to gradually return to training and sport, and the overall clinical picture generally guides clinicians.

Thoracic symptoms are less common, though progressive pain or deformity requires investigating. Plain films in this age group may show Scheuermann's kyphosis, in which three or more consecutive vertebrae show anterior wedging, postulated to result from abnormal end plate development in the upper thoracic spine or repetitive compressive forces more commonly in the lower thoracic spine, e.g. notably in gymnasts, rowers or footballers. Training load management and physiotherapy is important. Bracing may have a role in progressive cases or severe pain.

Scoliosis is a common finding on plain radiographs, but rarely causes pain, and is usually unrelated to sports participation.

MEDICAL MASQUERADES

There are certain important medical conditions that present as sport injuries due to a link the child has made to an accident or injury. A high level of suspicion is required not to miss these, particularly sinister causes in which a delay to diagnosis would be detrimental.

Inflammatory disease may first present to a clinician with low back pain and stiffness or tendon insertion pain (enthesopathy). A thorough history may reveal associated eye, skin, genitourinary or abdominal symptoms that require exclusion of a seronegative arthropathy. Diurnal pattern of the pain, such as early morning stiffness, often easing with movement can provide a key clue. Duration of stiffness can indicate severity.

Back pain or an apparent abdominal muscle strain may also be a presenting feature of intra-abdominal pathology such as ovarian cyst, inflammatory bowel disease or renal disease. These require exclusion via clinical assessment.

Childhood musculoskeletal tumours, such as sarcomas, often have a delay to diagnosis, particularly, in the early stages when red flag signs and symptoms such as night pain are absent. It is important to ensure that there is an accurate causal relationship between the putative mechanism of injury and the subsequent pain or disability and accurately correlate examination findings in order not to miss malignancy.

'Growing pains' are a diagnosis of exclusion via thorough history and examination. The pain usually affects the legs between the thighs and claves. The exact aetiology is unknown. The child is able to participate in PA without exacerbation. Mild-to-moderate night pain is a common feature, though eased by a trial of simple analgesics, stretching or massage. The child should be reviewed and investigated with plain radiographs, if there is any diagnostic doubt.

CHILD PROTECTION IN SPORT

Medical staff responsible for children should be aware of the possibility of abuse. All types of abuse may occur in the sporting environment, although neglect and emotional, physical and sexual abuse may be the most important of this environment.

It is emotional abuse that is often ignored in sport. Parental behaviours that ignore the child's wishes, undermine the child's performance or constitute verbal abuse of officials in front of children are all forms of abuse and need to be recognised and acted upon. All institutions involved in sport must have safeguarding policies and clearly identified staff responsible for child protection.

All staff working in the sporting environment should not put themselves in a position where allegations of sexual abuse could be made. It is an environment where children may be changing and showering and staff should be aware that children may feel vulnerable during this period.

Medical staff are also in a position to identify physical abuse. They should all be trained in child protection, and must be aware of factors suggesting following nonaccidental injuries:

- Delay in presentation
- Recurrent unexplained injury
- Unusual pattern of injury
- Withdrawn child
- Hiding injuries

All staff involved in the care or coaching of children are required to undergo enhanced screening from the Disclosure Barring Service in the United Kingdom.

CONCLUSION

The health benefits of exercise and the longer-term effects of inactivity are being increasingly recognised. Exercise and sport have a role to play in the management of a number of LTCs, imparting biopsychosocial health benefits. All health care practitioners must be encouraging patients to participate in PA, especially so children, to promote life-long positive health behaviours.

As more children take part in sport and exercise, injuries will occur and it is important that health care practitioners involved in the care of children are able to recognise the often more subtle features of injuries among children, and understand the need for appropriate management.

> **Key points for clinical practice**
>
> - All health care professionals should be promoting the benefits of exercise to children.
> - All health care professionals involved in the care of children should recognise the more subtle features of injuries in children.
> - Health care professionals should be careful not to miss serious pathology which may be mistaken for an injury.

REFERENCES

1. Brooks F, Magnusson J, Klemera E, et al. HBSC England national report: health behaviour in school-aged children (HBSC): World Health Organization collaborative cross national study. Hatfield; University of Hertfordshire, 2011.
2. Craig R, Mindell J, Hirani V. Health survey for England 2008; Volume 1, Physical activity and fitness. London: NHS Information Centre, 2009.
3. World Health Organization (WHO). Mortality and burden of disease attributable to selected major risks. In: Global health risks. Geneva: WHO Press, 2009.
4. British Heart Foundation National Centre (BHFNC). Economic costs of physical inactivity. Loughborough; BHFNC,2013.
5. Centre for Economics and Business Research (CEBR). The inactivity time bomb. London: CEBR, 2014.
6. Department of Health. At least five a week: Evidence on the impact of physical activity and its relationship to health – A report from the Chief Medical Officer, Crown Copyright. London: Department of Health, 2004.
7. Grontved A, Hu FB. Television viewing and risk of type 2 diabetes, cardiovascular disease, and all-cause mortality: a meta-analysis. JAMA 2011; 305:2440–2447.
8. Chau JY, Grunseit A, Midthjell K, et al. Cross-sectional associations of total sitting and leisure screen time with cardiometabolic risk in adults. Results from the HUNT Study, Norway. J Sci Med Sport 2014; 17:78–84.
9. Fereday J, MacDougall C, Spizzo M, et al. "There's nothing I can't do – I just put my mind to anything and I can do it": a qualitative analysis of how children with chronic disease and their parents account for and manage physical activity. BMC Pediatr 2009; 9:1.
10. Welsh L, Kemp JG, Roberts RG. Effects of physical conditioning on children and adolescents with asthma. Sports Med 2005; 35:127–141.
11. Dubow JS, Kelly JP. Epilepsy in sports and recreation. Sports Med 2003; 33:499–516.
12. van Camp SP, Bloor CM, Mueller FO, et al. Nontraumatic sports death in high school and college athletes. Med Sci Sports Exerc 1995; 27:641–647.
13. Pelliccia A, Fagard R, Bjornstad H, et al. Recommendations for competitive sports participation in athletes with cardiovascular disease: a consensus document from the Study Group of Sports Cardiology of the Working Group of Cardiac Rehabilitation and Exercise Physiology and the Working Group of Myocardial and Pericardial Diseases of the European Society of Cardiology. Eur Heart J 2005; 26:1422–1245.
14. Bongers B, van Brussell M, Hulzebos H, et al. Paediatric exercise testing in clincis and classrooms: a comparative review of different assessments. OA Epidemiol 2013; 1:14.
15. Department of Health, Physical Activity, Health Improvement and Protection. Start active, stay active: a report on physical activity from the four home countries' Chief Medical Officers. London: Department of Health, 2011.
16. Chief Medical Officer. Annual Report of the Chief Medical Officer 2012, Our Children Deserve Better: Prevention Pays. London: Department of Health, 2013.
17. Telama R, Yang X, Viikari J, et al. Physical activity from childhood to adulthood: a 21-year tracking study. Am J Prev Med 2005; 28:267–273.
18. Davis G, Purcell L. The evaluation and management of acute concussion differs in young children. Br J Sports Med 2014; 48:98–101.
19. De Maio V, Joseph D, Tibbo-Valeriote H, et al. Variability in discharge instructions and activity restrictions for patients evaluated in a childrens emergency department following concussion. Br J Sports Med 2012; 30:20–25.

20 Purcell L. What are the most appropriate return-to-play guidelines for concussed child athletes? Br J Sports Med 2009; 43:i51–i55.
21 Browne G, Lam LT. Concussive head injury in children and adolescents related to sports and other leisure physical activities. Br J Sports Med 2006; 40:163–168.
22 Maffuli N, Pintore E. Intensive training in young athletes. Br J Sports Med 1990; 24:237–239.
23 MacKelvie K, Khan K, McKay H. Is there a critical period for bone response to weight-bearing exercise in childrena nd adolscents? A systematic review. Br J Sports Med 2002; 36:250–257.
24 Caine D, DiFiori J, Maffulli N. Physeal Injuries in children's youth sport: reasons for concern? Br J Sports Med 2006; 40:749–760.
25 Behringer M, von Heede A, Yue Z, et al. Effects of resistance traiing in children and adolscents: a meta-analysis. Pediatrics 2010; 126:1199–1210.
26 Price R, Hawkins R, Hulse M, et al. The football association medical research programme: an audit of injuries in academy youth football. Br J Sports Med 2004; 38:466–471.
27 Oravo s, Virtanen K. Osteochondroses in athletes. Br J Sports Med 1982; 16:161–168.
28 Sailly M, Whiteley R, Johnson A. Doppler ultrasound and tibial tuberosity maturation status predicts pain in adolescent male athletes with Osgood–Schlatters disease: a case series with comparison group and clinical interpretation. Br J Sports Med 2013; 47:93–97.
29 Jones M, Straton G, Reilly T, et al. Biological risk indicators for recurrent non-specific low back pain in adolescents. Br J Sports Med 2005; 39:137–140.
30 Standaert C, Herring SA. Sponylolysis: a critical review. Br J Sports Med 2000; 34:415–422.

Chapter 4

Paediatric simulation training

Gabrielle Nuthall, Patricia Wood, Michael Shepherd

BACKGROUND

'Simulation is a technique – not a technology – to replace or amplify real experiences with guided experiences that evoke or replicate substantial aspects of the real world in a fully interactive manner' [1].

The traditional apprenticeship educational model of 'see one, do one, teach one' has been questioned as the best model for medical education and the use of simulation; both high and low fidelity has become common place in pediatric training in many institutions around the world. Simulation is especially useful in acute pediatrics as it offers methods for training staff in high-risk and often low-frequency events in children. Simulation allows the educator to plan in advance what skills the trainee needs to have and to learn and practise these without putting patients at risk.

Simulation is a multifaceted tool that can target teaching of technical skills, such as task trainers for insertion and taping of lines through to more difficult skills such as endotracheal intubation, right through to complex real-life multidisciplinary team training scenarios using high-fidelity computerised mannequins, such as placing an infant in cardiac arrest onto extra corporeal life support. It can also be targeted towards improving and/or testing systems performance.

Each simulation needs to take into account the needs of the learner, the participant mix, the simulator, the level of fidelity to be used, the environment and the educational objectives. Once decided upon these, the simulation can be planned in a variety of ways to achieve the educational aims and objectives.

A recent large systematic review and meta-analysis [2] reviewed the literature in terms of the effectiveness of simulation training for resuscitation training. The infrequency of cardiac arrest events limits the exposure on the job training and the critical nature of the event lends emergency resuscitation well to the use of simulation. This well-executed meta-analysis of 114 studies indicated that simulation training was highly effective. The additional features of the availability of 'booster' training sessions or practice sessions, team training and debriefing also improved effectiveness.

Gabrielle Nuthall MBChB FRACP FCICM, Paediatric Intensive Care Unit, Starship Children's Hospital, University of Auckland, Auckland, New Zealand. Email: GabrielleN@adhb.govt.nz (for correspondence)

Patricia Wood RGON PGDip, Children's Emergency Department and Simulation for Child Health, Starship Children's Hospital, University of Auckland, Auckland, New Zealand

Michael Shephard MBCHB FRACP MPH, Children's Emergency Department, Starship Children's Hospital, University of Auckland, Auckland, New Zealand

The suggestion in this meta-analysis that 'booster' session and debriefing from instructors enhance the value from simulation training is further supported by a recent study of Sutton et al [3] where they showed that brief bedside booster cardiopulmonary resuscitation (CPR) training, using instructors and automated defibrillator feedback, resulted in excellent quality CPR and improved knowledge retention in comparison to traditional teaching. Greater than 75% of participants achieved excellent CPR at the end of the study and >65% still performed excellent CPR before their final 6-month prebooster training, despite the short time the training took (a total of 20 minutes, with 5 minutes for each session).

While there are numerous articles, such as these, to be found in the literature supporting the use of simulation, the translation to actual improvement in patient outcomes is much more difficult to find and as yet is lacking in the literature. However, one group has demonstrated a suggestion of improvement in quality of patient care using simulation-based education. An academic teaching hospital used a retrospective case controlled study to compare residents who had received simulation-based education compared to those who had had advanced life support training with no simulation. During actual advanced cardiac life support (ACLS) resuscitation events, the residents with simulation-based training showed significantly higher adherence to American Heart Association (AHA) algorithms than the nonsimulation-trained residents (68% versus 48%), showing that the simulation-based health care had resulted in a significant improvement to quality of care received by the patients during the actual ACLS event [4].

SIMULATION CENTRES VERSUS IN SITU SIMULATION

Simulation teaching can either occur in dedicated facilities designed to replicate the patient care environment, either within the hospital or at an off-site location, a 'simulation centre', or simulation may occur within the hospital in the setting where patient care would typically occur, 'in-situ simulation'.

Historically, simulation started in simulation centres and is now more commonly found to be occurring in situ, but there are advantages and disadvantages of each, and both have their place depending upon the educational needs and aims of the learners as well as the teachers.

Setting up a dedicated simulation centre has implications upon cost, fidelity and access to simulation as it may be difficult for staff to get significant time away from work. Off-site simulation means separation from clinical responsibilities, thus, providing the benefit of uninterrupted training; however, this often requires the creation of ad-hoc teams from different hospitals or different parts of the hospital. Thus, some realism is lost and there may be difficulties in training native teams.

The other advantages of in-situ simulation are that staff do not have to be taken away from their normal environment and less time is taken away from actual patient care. Training occurs in their 'normal' environment, leading to the development of greater familiarity with local resources and equipment and as the environment is familiar it leads to greater realism (fidelity) of the simulation, making the teaching more valuable. Training is occurring with actual native clinical teams which facilitate the development of teamwork.

Training in-situ can also be used to identify latent safety threats within the health care environment, as described in more detail, later in this chapter.

However, in a busy clinical environment it can be busy to find space to run a simulation; attention needs to be paid to explaining to families what is happening if they are going to be exposed to simulated events (although this can actually make families feel safer to know that staff practice for emergencies). Simulation staff have to ensure there is minimal disruption and that staff who are working do not feel they are missing out on training.

The cost of setting up a whole simulation centre may be prohibitive for some hospitals and for those who prefer the advantages of in-situ simulation, one alternative that provides simulation at point of care is a mobile simulation cart. Weinstock et al [5] describe the use of and set up of a low space mobile simulation cart used to provide realistic simulation experiences to a wide range of groups within a hospital or within their normal working environment.

SIMULATION FOR SKILLS TRAINING

Learning theorists have long debated the various principles and methodology associated with adult education. Benner, Lieb, Dale and Knowles all concur that the historical approach to education must transition to a blended and more active model to engage the learner [6-9]. Simulation is an effective tool to teach and advance clinical skills. It allows for deliberative and repeated practice, using task trainers or low-fidelity mannequins in a safe and controlled setting, as clinicians develop and advance their clinical skills [7,10,11]. Simulation provides a realistic and active learning opportunity not possible in the classroom, at the same time eliminating risk to patients and staff [12-14]. A blended model of simulation and theoretical knowledge allows the learner to critically apply new knowledge to practice, in a safe environment and gain competence in a skill prior to transitioning to the bedside [14].

Health-like education is not static, and the scope of clinical expertise required of health professionals is constantly growing. The challenge for health professionals is to master and develop expertise utilising new and innovative technology, and to maintain mastery of skills over time.

Education of clinical skills requires consultation and planning; not every clinician can be expected to master every skill, so applicability to practice is an important consideration. The clinical skill set requirement varies according to role, scope and clinical setting, so learning must be structured accordingly to meet individual's need [8]. It is also important to acknowledge that it is not only novice practitioners who require new skills, but experienced clinicians also have to develop new skills and refresh current skills to ensure practice is up to the minute and they are adequately prepared to utilise new and innovative technology. The difference is that experienced clinicians have more depth of experience to augment their learning.

Categorisation of clinical skills is a strategy that can assist in determining education plans and methodology of teaching. Core, basic, everyday skills and frequently used skills such as auscultation, measuring vital signs will require a different approach to advanced, complex skills, infrequently used and critical skills [10,15].

Departments may use skills training to target specific areas that have been identified as needing improvement. An example of this is the targeting of improved delivery of time to deliver resuscitation fluids to children in shock in a busy children's emergency department [16]. Clinicians reported difficulty in the preparation and use of fluid delivery equipment. The methodology of fluid delivery was analysed; best practice was established and retaught to nurses, using in-situ equipment and environment. Performance and confidence were observed and measured, with improvement in all but one individual (**Figure 4.1**). Skill refresher training in rapid fluid administration improved the performance of nurses who had identified a gap in their practice and were willing participants of an innovative competitive approach. Friendly competition provided incentive to participate in skill-refresher training. Regular training is likely to be required to maintain efficiency in skills that are used infrequently.

CPR is a widely studied skill and while used infrequently, effective chest compressions can be the difference between life with or without neurological impairment, and death. Maintaining compliance with CPR training (**Figure 4.2**) is an ongoing requirement which has inherent challenges. Despite regular updates, studies have demonstrated that health professionals often demonstrate inadequate CPR skills [17]. A novel approach was instigated by Niles [17] using just-in-time and just-in-place teaching, where skills training occurred in the clinical setting for brief skills update. This resulted in significantly shorter times to achieve proficient CPR skills.

Moore [11] also studied the high-risk, low-volume clinical skill of fibre-optic intubation (FOI). Anaestheology has led the way in the use of simulation in health education,

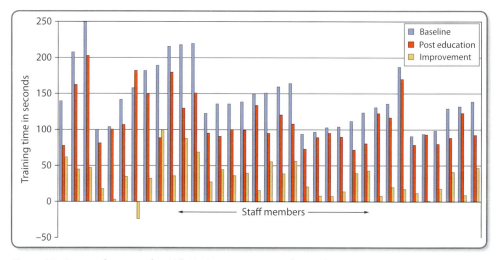

Figure 4.1 Nurse performance of rapid fluid administration pre and post education.

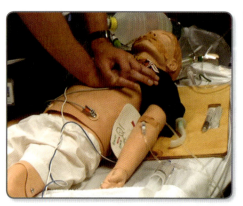

Figure 4.2 Cardiopulmonary resuscitation skills training.

as practising intubation on an awake patient would lead to harm. Participants used a multimodal approach including a didactic lecture, a step-by-step guide followed by a series of three FOI on a high-fidelity manikin. This allowed for deliberate and repeat practice and engagement in skills not readily available in the classroom or in everyday practice. Results showed a significant decrease in time of FOI following training and practice.

Simulation for skills training is becoming a mainstream in the health profession. However, using Waxman's [9] parallel to aviation, it is important to acknowledge that just as pilots, it is unacceptable for a trainee pilot to move from flying in a simulator to captaining a passenger jet, health professionals need to transition skills from simulation to the bedside using a measured approach.

SIMULATION AND TEAM TRAINING

In the early 1990s, a group led by David Gaba at Stanford University advocated simulation-based training in the management of anaesthesia crises, using crew resource management principles from aviation [18-20]. This approach is now widely known as crisis resource management (CRM) training and has spread to be used internationally to train health care teams across a broad range of medical specialties and of different levels of expertise. The identified benefits of multidisciplinary simulation-based CRM training are a lack of patient risk and efficient and scheduled use of training time. This helps the teams to learn and practise the work place skills and behaviours required to manage rare or hazardous clinical events by placing the adult learner in an authentic environment [21].

CRM training teaches skills in teamwork and communication with the five main principles of CRM being role clarity, communication, personnel support, resource use and global assessment. Emphasis is placed on the practical application of these principles within the clinical environment where the course is being held. A specific and detailed description of this is well described by Allen et al [22] in the paediatric cardiac intensive care unit, along with encouraging results, showing decreased anxiety among multidisciplinary team members and increased preparedness for future real-life crisis events.

Paediatric resuscitation and acute medical care are unique. A different set of skills are required in the resuscitation of children, e.g. medication calculation, equipment selection, use of different resuscitation algorithms and technical skills (e.g. airway management and intraosseous insertion). Life-threatening emergencies such as cardiac arrest are also less common than in adults, so the combination of different skills being required and infrequent events makes paediatric acute medical emergencies an ideal situation for CRM training. Teamwork during resuscitation is not well studied, but it has been shown to be suboptimal and the absence of both leadership and task distribution can adversely effect the translation of theoretical knowledge into effective team management of patients [23].

The importance of the initiation of high quality CPR is well documented and there is evidence that the delivery of high-quality CPR could be improved upon. Hunt et al [24] prospectively studied the first 5 minutes of paediatric mock codes in the ward setting. They assessed time taken for specific resuscitation manoeuvers to occur, team behaviours and adherence to AHA basic life support algorithms. They found alarming delays in initiation of appropriate interventions: 75% of simulated resuscitated events deviated from AHA guidelines and 100% had a communication error occured. Studies such as these give weight to the importance of team training attempting to improve the quality of CPR by targeting these areas.

CRM training (**Figure 4.2**) is well suited to attempt to address these issues, especially within the unique challenges faced by paediatric practitioners.

SIMULATION AND SAFETY IMPROVEMENT IN PAEDIATRICS

In-situ training using simulation has been used to identify latent safety threats in the health care environment. Latent safety threats are errors in the design of the environment, organisation or maintenance that are found to have potential impact on the delivery of health care and patient safety. Simulation has a role to play in both new health care developments and the testing and improvement of existing environments with increasing literature describing these benefits across a range of clinical areas. Identification of these errors and issues requires a systematic approach to the delivery of simulation-based training, with a post-training debrief being used to identify any significant clinical issues and determine how they will be reported to departmental/organisation leadership.

In the perinatal environment, several programmes of in-situ simulation have reported successful identification of latent environmental threats to patient safety [25,26]. The most extensive of these was able to demonstrate a significant benefit of in-situ training across a range of locations [26]. This programme used a set of standardised scenarios based on previous sentinel events and used a defensive barrier safety model to identify a range of active and latent safety breaches. An example is shown in **Figure 4.3** of a young child with a post tonsillectomy bleed which is being used for in situ simulation teaching.

In neonatology, a multidisciplinary-team-training programme using in-situ simulation identified an average of 1.8 latent safety threats per scenario [27]. Owing to integration with departmental leadership, this programme was able to demonstrate objective clinical improvements following the identification of these safety threats.

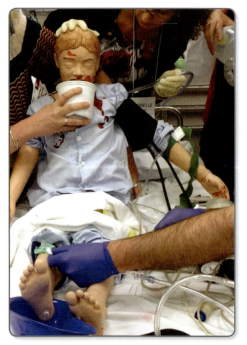

Figure 4.3 Emergency department crisis resource management of child with tonsillar bleed.

In the emergency department (ED) setting, short unannounced simulations were able to identify approximately one latent safety threat per simulation [28]. Of note, participants generally felt satisfied with the experience, with little clinical impact identified by staff. It was suggested that the regularity and high frequency of these events assisted with staff engagement.

In the paediatric ward setting, a similar unannounced in-situ simulation methodology has been described [29]. This programme identified a large number of latent safety threats around the hospital and a range of personal knowledge gaps and CRM skills among staff. Another ward-based in-situ simulation programme has reported identification of important latent safety threats [30].

Identification of latent safety errors and potential solutions should be significant drivers for the establishment and maintenance of multidisciplinary simulation-based training in health-care organisations. The patient safety improvements and other efficiencies that follow from such programmes are now well recognised. More traditional safety systems are reactive and ad hoc, waiting for relatively infrequent sentinel events to generate an investigation looking for generalisable problems. Simulation has been demonstrated to deliver safety improvements in a more systematic and robust manner. The hallmark of these successful programmes is the use of multidisciplinary teams, in high-fidelity simulation, with a clear mechanism for reporting safety threats and acting to eliminate them [31].

SIMULATION FOR ASSESSMENT IN PAEDIATRICS

There are a range of theoretical reasons why simulation may be a suitable tool for the assessment of practitioner competency and subsequent credentialing, training and quality improvement. Simulation may allow for assessment of more complex core competencies, especially those involving dynamic interactions, e.g. procedural skills and professionalism. Simulation may increase the validity of assessment outcome by replicating the environment and complexity of real clinical paediatric setting. Simulation will offer an error-tolerant and safe environment to complete assessments, as well as providing much greater control over assessment content. By contrast, many clinical examinations are dependent on availability of suitable patients.

The evaluation of validity of an assessment has been detailed in the US Standards for Educational and Psychological Testing [32], with content validity, inter-rater reliability, internal structure of scoring, external validity and potential consequences of the assessment process, all being important components. A recent review of simulation-based assessment of health professionals was completed by Cook et al [33]. This showed that among 417 published studies, 84% involved physicians and most involved skills assessment for CPR or surgical skills. Validity assessment was infrequently carried out according to these standards and reporting was not systematic [32].

SKILLS ASSESSMENT

With regard to skills assessment using simulation, some important principles can be established from the existing literature. Firstly, it is unlikely that simulation-based assessment will be suitable as the only method of assessment. While few studies have directly compared assessment techniques, Nunnink assessed intensive care trainees' ability to manage a blocked tracheostomy using written examination, simulation-based and oral viva examinations [34]. They demonstrated low correlation between written examination and oral viva or simulation. Of particular note was that a proportion of trainees who passed the written examination performed a number of dangerous errors in simulation, thus suggesting that multimodal assessment is likely to be required.

Secondly, when developing scoring systems, a global assessment score is an essential addition to a checklist-based scoring system. Ma et al used a checklist to assess video-recorded simulated central venous catheter insertion and found that while a checklist score of <80% was a strong indication of incompetence, a high checklist score did not preclude incompetence [35]. Ratings using a global rating scale identified an additional 32% of candidates who committed serious errors (and, thus, were deemed incompetent) despite scoring well on the checklists.

Thirdly, the assessment is likely to be more discriminatory if it includes qualitative measures of skills achievement and allows for demonstration of a whole procedure. For example, in the assessment of laparoscopic cholecystectomy, 'dissection accuracy' was associated with greater experience and skill but only the full procedure showed complete discrimination between the expert and novice [36].

Features of good skills assessment include the following:
1. Presence of a skills trainer with adequate fidelity to replicate the physical performance of the task
2. Developed measures that have content validity
3. Have a global rating score and use a checklist
4. Measure more than simple achievement of physical steps, include a qualitative element, e.g.:
   i. Time to achieve task (in a time critical task)
   ii. Strength of knot
   iii. Position of chest tube

ASSESSMENT OF MORE COMPLEX COMPETENCIES

The assessment of more complex competencies using simulation has been led by the field of anaesthesia. Simulation has been used to assess resident competency across a range of domains, in a range of clinical scenarios [37,38]. This work demonstrates that assessment can be developed with reliability and validity. However, further work is required to match this assessment process with clinically observed competency and comma across a range of other disciplines.

A number of tools have been developed that will assist in the development of simulation-based assessments of more complex competencies. The 'simulation module for assessment of resident targeted event responses' approach was designed to assist with the development of emergency medicine trainee assessment. However, it has a broad applicability, providing a systematic method for creating simulation-based scenarios and measurement tools [39]. This tool emphasises linking to overall objectives, focussing scenarios on fairly narrow areas, using multiple assessments (sampling), being specific about what the 'good' looks like and designing and mapping scenarios to match this.

Even more complex competencies are team based and there is little definitive evidence base for the use of simulation for assessment in this area. A comprehensive methodology has been reported to assist with building simulation-based team assessments – 'DEEP' (distinguish, elaborate, establish and proceduralise) [40]; however, further research is required to validate the output from such an approach.

There is very little evidence about the acceptability of simulation-based assessment to those being assessed. Anecdotal experience suggests that it can be acceptable; however, concerns have been raised about the possibility of simulation-based assessment reducing the safety of simulation-based education. In a small study of critical care trainees, simulation-based assessment was acceptable to the trainees [41].

In summary, the use of simulation for assessment in paediatrics (and in health care generally) has an increasing evidence base, but some limitations and caveats have been identified. Assessment is likely to be most reliable if more than one modality is utilised (e.g. written examination and simulation) and global scoring systems and checklists are combined. It is clear that careful planning is required to identify objectives, develop simulation-based experiences, develop scoring systems and standardise scenario delivery. Simulation-based assessment is likely to be time consuming, requires simulation delivery experience and skill, and a safe delivery methodology for students (including previous simulation experience and detailed orientation).

Further work is required to develop a wider research base around the valid assessment of more complex skills and professional competencies and to further assess the acceptability of this methodology.

CONCLUSION

The advantages of simulation training facilitated by experienced instructors are that it:
- allows practice in a risk-free environment;
- facilitates reflective learning for the adult learner;
- allows skill to be practiced repeatedly
- provides on-demand learning with exposure to both common and high-risk uncommon clinical situation;
- allows the ability to evaluate and teach the use of new protocols, new equipment, new clinical areas; facilitates multidisciplinary team training;
- assists with the detection and amelioration of latent safety threats, therefore, reducing medical error; and
- is a modality that allows for the assessment of more complex competencies.

Its use is increasingly supported by a large body of literature, both across many specialties of medicine and levels of expertise right through from medical students to expert practitioners. It is especially pertinent to paediatric practice because of the challenges faced with decreased clinical exposure to infrequent critical events, the increasingly unacceptable nature of 'practicing upon children' and the nature of paediatric practice where a wide range of different sized children and clinical problems are faced by clinicians on a regular basis.

Key points for clinical practice

- Simulation as an educational tool is helpful to all levels of experience in healthcare, not just the novice learner.
- Simulation education must be carefully planed, measured and audited, to ensure the it achieves the intended objectives and to be successful.
- Simulation is a powerful tool, not only for teaching of clinical skills, but also to improve team training, safety of hospital systems and potentially for assessment of clinical competencies.

REFERENCES

1. Gaba DM. The future vision of simulation in healthcare. Qual Saf Health Care 2004; 13:i2–i10.
2. Mundell WC, Kennedy CC, Szostek JH, et al. Simulation technology for resuscitation technology: a systematic review and meta-analysis. Resuscitation 2013; 84:1174–1183.
3. Sutton RM, Niles D, Meaney PA, et al. Low-dose, high-frequency CPR training improves skill retention of in-hospital pediatric providers. Pediatrics 2011; 128:e145–e151.
4. Wayne DB, Didwania A, Feinglass J, et al. Simulation-based education improves quality of care during cardiac arrest team responses at an academic teaching hospital. A case –control study. Chest 2008; 133:56–61.
5. Weinstock PH, Kappus LJ, Garden A, et al. Simulation at the point of care; reduced-cost, in situ training via a mobile cart. Pediatr Crit Care Med 2009; 10:176–182.
6. Benner P. From novice to expert: excellence and power in clinical nursing practice. Menlo Park, CA: Addison-Wesley, 1984.
7. Kneebone R. Evaluating clinical simulations for learning procedural skills: a theory based approach. Acad Med 2005; 80:6.
8. Rennie I. Exploring approaches to clinical skills development in nursing education. Nurs Times 2009; 105: 20–22.
9. Waxman KT, Telles CL. The use of Benner's framework in high-fidelity simulation faculty development. The Bay area simulation collaborative model. Clin Simul Nurs 2009; 5:e231–e235.
10. Ericsson K. Deliberate practice and acquisition of expert performance: a general overview. Acad Emerg Med 2008; 15:988–994.
11. Moore K, Smith S, Curry D, et al. Simulation training for fiber-optic intubations. Clin Simul Nurs , 2014; 10:470–475.
12. Gonzalez L, Sole M. Urinary catheterization skills: one simulated checkoff is not enough. Clin Simul Nurs , (2014; 10:455–460.
13. Ross J. Simulation and psychomotor skill acquisition: a review of the literature. Clin Simul Nurs (2012; 8:e429–e3435.
14. White A, Brannan J, Long J, et al. Comparison of instructional methods: cognitive skills and confidence levels. Clin Simul Nurs 2013; 9:417–423.
15. Scalese R, Obese V, Issenberg S. Simulation technology for skills training and competency assessment in medical education. J Gen Intern Med 2007; 23:46–49.
16. Wood T, Hollis S, Dalziel S. et al. Use of multi-modal simulation to improve fluid resuscitation in a pediatric emergency department. Poster presentation International pediatric simulation symposia and workshops, New York, 2013.
17. Niles D, Sutton R, Donoghue A, et al. 'Rolling refreshers': A novel approach to maintain CPR psychomotor skill competence. Resuscitation 2009; 80:909–912.
18. Billings CE, Reynard WD. Human factors in aircraft incidents: results of a 7-year study. Aviat Space Environ Med 1984; 55:960–965.
19. Cooper GE, White MD, Lauber JK. Resource Management on the Flightdeck: Proceedings of a NASA/Industry Workshop. (NASA CP-2120). Moffett Field, CA: NASA-Ames Research Center, 1980.
20. Howard SK, Gaba DM, Fish KJ, et al. Anesthesia crisis resource management training: teaching anesthesiologists to handle critical incidents. Aviat Space Environ Med 1992; 63:763–770.
21. Aldrich C. Learning by doing: a comprehensive guide to simulations, computer games, and pedagogy in e-learning and other educational experiences. San Francisco, CA: Pfieffer, 2005.
22. Allen CK, Thiagarajan RR, Beke D, et al. Simulation-based training delivered directly to the pediatric cardiac intensive care unit engenders preparedness, comfort, and decreased anxiety among multidisciplinary resuscitation team members. J Thorac Cardiovasc Surg 2010; 140:646–652.
23. Marsch SCU, Muller C, Marquardt K, et al. Human factors affect the quality of cardiopulmonary resuscitation in simulated cardiac arrests. Resuscitation 2004; 60:51–56.
24. Hunt EA, Walker AR, Shaffner DH, et al. Simulation of in-hospital pediatric medical emergencies and cardiopulmonary arrests: highlighting the importance of the first 5 minutes. Pediatrics 2008; 121:e34–e43.
25. Hamman WR, Beaudin-Seiler BM, Beaubien JM, et al. Using in situ simulation to identify and resolve latent environmental threats to patient safety: case study involving operational changes in a labor and delivery ward. Qual Manag Health Care 2010; 19:226–230.

26. Riley W, Davis S, Miller KM, et al. Detecting breaches in defensive barriers using in situ simulation for obstetric emergencies. Qual Saf Health Care 2010; 19:i53–i56.

27. Wetzel EA, Lang TR, Pendergrass TL, et al. Identification of latent safety threats using high-fidelity simulation-based training with multidisciplinary neonatology teams. Jt Comm J Qual Patient Saf 2013; 39:268–273.

28. Patterson MD, Geis GL, Falcone RA, et al. In situ simulation: detection of safety threats and teamwork training in a high risk emergency department. BMJ Qual Saf 2013; 22:468–477.

29. Wheeler DS, Geis G, Mack EH, et al. High-reliability emergency response teams in the hospital: improving quality and safety using in situ simulation training. BMJ Qual Saf 2013; 22:507–514.

30. Garden AL, Mills SA, Wilson R, et al. In situ simulation training for paediatric cardiorespiratory arrest: initial observations and identification of latent errors. Anaesth Intensive Care 2010; 38:1038–1042.

31. Guise JM, Mladenovic J. In situ simulation: identification of systems issues. Semin Perinatol 2013; 37:161–165.

32. American Educational Research Association (AERA), American Psychological Association, National Council of Measurement in Education. Standards for educational and psychological testing. Washington, DC: AERA, 2014.

33. Cook DA, Brydges R, Zendejas B, et al. Technology-enhanced simulation to assess health professionals: a systematic review of validity evidence, research methods, and reporting quality. Acad Med 2013; 88:872–883.

34. Nunnink L, Venkatesh B, Krishnan A, et al. A prospective comparison between written examination and either simulation-based or oral viva examination of intensive care trainees' procedural skills. Anaesth Intensive Care 2010; 38:876–882.

35. Ma I, Zalunardo N, Pachev G, et al. Comparing the use of global rating scale with checklists for the assessment of central venous catheterization skills using simulation. Adv Health Sci Educ Theory Pract 2012; 17:457–470.

36. Van Bruwaene S, Schijven MP, Miserez M. Assessment of procedural skills using virtual simulation remains a challenge. J Surg Educ 2014; 71:654–661.

37. Blum RH, Boulet JR, Cooper JB, et al. Simulation-based assessment to identify critical gaps in safe anesthesia resident performance. Anesthesiology 2014; 120:129–141.

38. Fehr JJ, Boulet JR, Waldrop WB, et al. Simulation-based assessment of pediatric anesthesia skills. Anesthesiology 2011; 115:1308–1315.

39. Rosen MA, Salas E, Silvestri S, et al. A measurement tool for simulation-based training in emergency medicine: the simulation module for assessment of resident targeted event responses (SMARTER) approach. Simul Healthc 2008; 3:170–179.

40. Grand JA, Pearce M, Rench TA, et al. Going DEEP: guidelines for building simulation-based team assessments. BMJ Qual Saf 2013; 22:436–448.

41. Nunnink L, Foot C, Venkatesh B, et al. High-stakes assessment of the non-technical skills of critical care trainees using simulation: feasibility, acceptability and reliability. Crit Care Resusc 2014; 16:6–12.

Chapter 5

C-reactive protein and procalcitonin in assessment of children with fever in the emergency department

Ruud G Nijman, Alain Gervaix, Ian K Maconochie, Rianne Oostenbrink

INTRODUCTION

Fever is among the most common presenting symptoms in paediatric emergency care, contributing to 10–30% of consultations [1]. Children up to an age of 18 months have on average eight febrile episodes; in 20–40% of such cases, a professional health care provider is consulted [2]. Only a minority (7–15%) of febrile children has a serious bacterial infection (SBI) [3,4], with pneumonia and urinary tract infection (UTI) being the most frequent type of infections. The incidence of SBI, and, in particular, the occurrence of bacterial sepsis and meningitis, dropped markedly over the last few decades owing to the expansion of national vaccination schemes [5]. Yet, neither the number of febrile children visiting emergency care facilities nor parental help-seeking behaviour has changed [6]. Also, an increase in short-stay hospital admissions among children with acute infections was recently demonstrated [7]. Moreover, a significant number of febrile children continue to receive antibiotics that are unlikely to benefit them with the added effect of contributing to the development of antimicrobial resistance, while other children still succumb to treatable infectious diseases as a result of failure to recognise SBI at an early stage of the disease [8].

As clinical signs and symptoms are often of limited value in distinguishing SBI from self-limiting febrile illnesses [9], biomarkers, such as C-reactive protein (CRP) and procalcitonin (PCT), are often used for this purpose. This chapter provides an overview of the available studies on CRP and PCT as diagnostic markers in febrile children, and aims to guide physicians dealing with children with fever in secondary care on the use of CRP and PCT.

Ruud G Nijman MD PhD, Department of Paediatric Accident and Emergency, St. Mary's Hospital, London, UK. Email: r.g.nijman@erasmusmc.nl (for correspondence)

Alain Gervaix MD, Division of Paediatric Emergency, University Children's Hospital, Geneva, Switzerland

Ian K Maconochie FRCPCH FRCEM FRCPI PhD, Department of Paediatric Accident and Emergency, St. Mary's Hospital, London, UK

Rianne Oostenbrink MD PhD, Department of General Paediatrics, Erasmus MC, Sophia Children's Hospital, Rotterdam, The Netherlands

METHODS

A systematic research was conducted to identify papers on the topic of CRP and PCT as diagnostic tools in the diagnostic management of febrile children at the emergency department (ED). The search was performed in addition to a systematic search by the European Network on Recognising Serious Infections, the latter search having been published in 2011 [10]. The results of the composite systematic review have been published in early 2014 as part of the Dutch National Guideline for the management of febrile children in secondary care [11]. Additionally, for this chapter, the search was repeated to identify any relevant papers published after June 2012 up to August 2014.

Snowballing methodology and expert consensus by the authors was applied to identify any relevant papers on the topic not included in the original searches. Systematic reviews were preferred, and complemented by large observational studies or randomised trials published after the systematic review appeared in print. Primarily, papers comparing CRP and PCT were reviewed, but papers on a single biomarker were also considered.

INTERPRETING DIAGNOSTIC VALUES

The diagnostic value of a biomarker and its associated clinical usefulness are determined by its capacity to change clinical decision making, e.g. by influencing decisions for performing additional diagnostic tests or starting antibiotic treatment. Likelihood ratios (LRs) illustrate the change of a clinical risk estimate with a positive or negative test result taking the prior chance of having SBI into account. This pretest risk equates to the incidence of SBI in the population at risk, which is between 7% and 15% in most emergency care settings, with higher incidences, up to 25%, being reported [3,4,12]. **Figure 5.1** shows the effect that a positive or negative test has on the change in clinical risk. Generally, negative LRs <0.2 are viewed as strongly supportive for ruling out SBI, and positive LRs >5.0 for ruling in SBIs. The area under the receiver operating characteristic (ROC) curve is another measure of diagnostic performance that is commonly used. The ROC area resembles a nonparametric test, comparing a case and a noncase for each possible cut-off value with values between 0.5 and 1, with 0.5 resembling a noninformative test and 1 being a perfect discriminatory test [13]. Other frequently used measures of diagnostic performance are sensitivity, specificity and predictive values.

PHYSIOLOGY OF CRP AND PCT

CRP was first described in 1930 by Tillet and Francis [14]. They discovered a protein that precipitated with pneumococcal C-polysaccharide in patients with pneumococcal pneumonia. CRP is now known to be an acute phase protein secreted by the liver in response to tissue damage or inflammation. Its clinical use is advocated in a wide array of paediatric and adult diagnostic dilemmas. Increased levels of PCT in children with signs of systemic infection were first reported in the early 1990s by Assicot et al [15]. Earlier studies in adults had looked at PCT in medullary thyroid carcinoma and staphylococcal toxic shock syndrome [16]. PCT is a 116-aminoacid peptide and a precursor of calcitonin and is believed to be an amplifier of the inflammatory cascade [17]. Differences in protein kinetics between PCT and CRP result in earlier increased serum concentration levels of PCT than

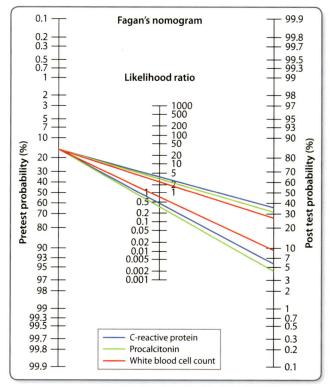

Figure 5.1 Fagan's nomogram. Changes in risk estimates using positive and negative likelihood ratios of a diagnostic test. In this instance, the pooled estimates as described by Yo et al are used [22], and an incidence of serious bacterial infections of 15%. In this nomogram it is clearly depicted how procalcitonin (PCT) has the best value for ruling out serious bacterial infection (SBI) and C-reactive protein (CRP) for ruling in SBI, and both CRP and PCT outperforming white blood cell count.

CRP levels [18-20]. For example, PCT could be detected in the plasma 2 hours after the intravenous injection of endotoxins, whereas CRP could be detected only after 12 hours. In addition, PCT concentration levels rose during the first 6–8 hours and reached a plateau after approximately 12 hours, before returning to normal concentration levels within 2–3 days. In contrast, CRP reached a plateau after 20–72 hours and decreased to normal values within 3–7 days [18-20].

CRP AND PCT AS SOLITARY MARKERS

Three systematic reviews were published on the diagnostic ability of CRP and PCT to identify SBI in febrile children (**Table 5.1**) [10,21,22]. Overall, the diagnostic performances of PCT and CRP were strikingly similar across the three systematic reviews. CRP and PCT were both useful for ruling in SBI in febrile children, as reflected by high positive LRs and specificities, and ruling out SBI, as reflected by high negative LRs and sensitivities. Yo et al claimed that PCT might be a better marker than CRP for ruling out SBI with slightly better sensitivities and negative LRs. However, in a subgroup analyses of the studies in emergency care settings CRP and PCT performed similarly. Van den Bruel et al proposed using a cut-off of 20 mg/L for CRP for ruling out SBI (range negative LR 0.19–0.25) and a cut-off of 80 mg/L for ruling in SBI [one study, positive LR 8,4, 95% confidence interval (CI): 5.1-14.1]. For PCT, they suggested using a cut-off of 0.5 ng/mL for ruling out SBI (range negative LR 0.08–0.25) and a cut-off of 2 ng/mL (two studies, range positive LR 3.6–13.7) for ruling in SBI.

Table 5.1 Diagnostic values of C-reactive protein, procalcitonin and white blood cell count for detecting serious bacterial infections in febrile children *							
Biomarkers	Population	No. of studies	Sensitivity (95% CI)	Specificity (95% CI)	Positive LR (95% CI)	Negative LR (95% CI)	ROC area (95% CI)
C-reactive protein							
Sanders et al [21]	Total	6	0.77 (0.68–0.83)	0.79 (0.74–0.83)	3.64 (2.99–4.43)	0.29 (0.22–0.40)	NA
Van den Bruel et al [10]	Total	5	0.75 (0.63–0.85)	0.76 (0.71–0.81)	3.15 (2.67–3.71). 2.40–3.79 (range)	0.33 (0.22–0.49) 0.25–0.61 (range)	NA
Yo et al [22]	Total	6	0.74 (0.65–0.82)	0.76 (0.70–0.81)	3.10 (2.48–3.87)	0.34 (0.25–0.46)	0.81 (0.78–0.84)
	Emergency care setting	4	0.75 (0.63–0.84)	0.80 (0.76–0.84)	3.82 (3.19–4.58)	0.35 (0.22–0.56)	0.84 (0.81–0.87)
	Age ≤ 36 months	4	0.75 (0.61–0.84)	0.75 (0.68–0.80)	2.90 (2.14–3.94)	0.31 (0.21–0.46)	0.81 (0.77 – 0.87)
Procalcitonin							
Van den Bruel et al [10]	Total	3	NA	NA	1.75–3.11 (range)	0.08–0.35 (range)	NA
Yo et al [22]	Total	8	0.83 (0.70–0.91)	0.69 (0.59–0.85)	2.69 (1.87–3.87)	0.25 (0.15 – 0.40)	0.84 (0.80–0.87)
	Emergency care settings	6	0.84 (0.69–0.93)	0.69 (0.51–0.83)	2.70 (1.75–4.18)	0.23 (0.13–0.41)	0.85 (0.81–0.87)
	Age ≤ 36 months	6	0.82 (0.71–0.90)	0.72 (0.63–0.80)	2.98 (2.20–4.05)	0.25 (0.15–0.41)	0.84 (0.81–0.87)
White blood cell count							
Van den Bruel et al [10]		7	NA	NA	0.87–2.43 (range)	0.61–1.14 (range)	NA
Yo et al [22]	Total	7	0.58 (0.49–0.67)	0.73 (0.67–0.77)	2.11 (1.63–2.74)	0.58 (0.46–0.73)	0.70 (0.65–0.74)
	Emergency care settings	5	0.59 (0.51–0.67)	0.76 (0.73–0.78)	2.48 (2.08–2.95)	0.53 (0.44–0.65)	0.77 (0.73–0.80)
	Age ≤ 36 months	6	0.58 (0.47–0.68)	0.71 (0.65–0.77)	2.09 (1.49–2.95)	0.58 (0.43 – 0.79)	0.70 (0.66–0.74)

*Pooled estimates or range.
CI, confidence interval; LR, likelihood ratio; NA, not applicable; ROC, receiver operating characteristic.

COMBINING CRP AND PCT IN PREDICTION MODELS

Neither CRP nor PCT is able to reliably rule out or rule in the presence of SBI by themselves. Combinations of biomarkers have been proposed, of which the so-called Lab-score is the one best known and most studied. The Lab score is based on univariate regression coefficients combined in an easy-to-use score consisting of CRP (<40, 40–99, or ≥100 mg/L), PCT (<0.5, 0.5 to <2, or ≥2 ng/mL) and abnormal urine dipstick (dipstick positive for nitrates and/or leukocytes) [26]. The initial study showed promising value for both ruling in and out SBI (score ≥3, positive LR 4.92, 95% CI 3.26–7.43, negative LR 0.07, 95% CI 0.02–0.27) [26], confirmed by a first validation study [12]. However, two validation studies showed good ability for ruling in SBI, but not so good for ruling out SBI [27,28]. A randomised controlled trial introducing the Lab-score to guide antibiotic prescribing was not useful in reducing prescribing rates in a paediatric ED, although a reduction could have been achieved safely by complying with Lab-score-associated recommendations [29].

Others have aimed to improve diagnostic ability by positioning CRP and PCT within the clinical context. In one validated prediction model, CRP in conjunction with clinical features proved to be a good predictor for having pneumonia as well as of having other types of SBI among which were UTI and septicaemia [4]. Importantly, including CRP gave a better prediction model than one just consisting of clinical features. The prediction model is available through the website www.erasmusmc.nl/feverkidstool and provides a risk estimate for the chance of having pneumonia or having another type of SBI. The same authors showed that adding PCT values only influenced clinical decision making in those children with intermediate values CRP (between 20 and 100 mg/L) in particular, which made up for less than one third of the population [28]. For solely, the prediction of bacterial pneumonia, CRP does not appear to be an important predictor. A systematic review including eight studies and 1230 children concluded only a weakly predictive effect of CRP (odds ratio 2.6, 95% CI 1.2–5.6) [30]. CRP has not been recommended for routine use in making the diagnosis of pneumonia in the guideline by the British Thoracic Society [31]. Contrastingly, a validated prediction model showed that CRP was useful in children at a clinical intermediate risk of pneumonia based on severity of illness, oxygen saturation and breathing rate [32].

SEQUENTIAL MEASUREMENTS OF PCT AND CRP

Several studies support the potential of serial levels of CRP and PCT in the paediatric ED. One study showed that children without SBI who had an early increase of CRP also had early stabilisation of CRP levels, whereas CRP levels in children with SBI continued to rise [33]. One of the few studies looking at serial PCT measurements in children visiting an ED described a randomised controlled trial among children suspected of a lower respiratory tract infection. In this study, children in the intervention arm underwent PCT testing at the ED, followed by PCT sampling on days 3 and 5. Results showed that the availability of PCT did not influence prescribing rate of antibiotics, but that it did reduce the duration for which antibiotics were given while there was no difference in return of daily activities between the PCT-guided and control patients [34]. Similarly, a randomised controlled trial, using a single PCT measure to guide physicians in their antibiotics, prescribing in a paediatric ED also did not show an effect on antibiotics prescribing, and showed that prophylactic use of antibiotics in children with high levels of PCT would lead to increased prescribing rates without effecting clinical outcomes [35]. Another randomised controlled trial looking at serial PCT measurements in hospitalised children with lower respiratory tract infections described that PCT resulted in lower antibiotics prescribing rates and shorter duration of antibiotics course. These findings comply with the conclusions of a Cochrane review in adults with suspected lower respiratory tract infections showing that serial measurements of PCT reduced the duration of antibiotics course without influencing morbidity and mortality [36]. As yet, there are no studies comparing the usefulness of serial measurements of CRP and PCT in febrile children in the ED.

CRP, PCT AND DURATION OF FEVER

It has been suggested PCT is a better marker than CRP to identify SBI in children with a short duration of fever. A study by Luaces-Cubells et al found PCT to be superior to CRP in infants with fever of <8 hours duration (ROC area 0.97 for PCT and 0.76 for CRP). Similarly, Olaciregui et al concluded that PCT was more useful than CRP in young febrile infants aged <3 months with an onset of fever <12 hours [37]. However, the limited number of children with SBI who had a short onset of fever in both studies should be taken into account when interpreting those findings. Nijman et al found that the duration of fever, with a cut-off point of 24 hours, did not influence the diagnostic performance of PCT or CRP [28]. Pratt et al showed that the diagnostic value of CRP in children with a fever lasting >12 hours was better than in children with a short onset of fever (ROC area 0.92 versus 0.68) [19], similar to the conclusions of Segal et al [33].

CRP AND PCT IN YOUNG FEBRILE INFANTS

An observational study by Gomes et al in 1112 well-appearing young febrile infants (up to an age of 3 months) found PCT to be a better marker than CRP for identifying infants with an invasive bacterial infection, i.e. proven bacterial sepsis or meningitis [38]. However, CRP and PCT showed similar predictive ability for identifying any type of SBI. In this study, 289 (26%) children had SBI with 23 (2%) children having an invasive bacterial infection. Supporting the generalisability of their findings, this study was conducted across seven European emergency care departments; on the other hand, they used a selected population, only including those infants who had a blood culture taken. In the same cohort of young febrile infants, another study looked into the validity of the Lab-score [27]. In this instance, the predictive ability for detecting invasive bacterial infections was similar to that of predicting any SBI, indicating that the Lab-score was more useful for ruling in than for ruling out SBI and invasive bacterial infections. Using the Lab-score would have misdiagnosed 7 (30%) infants with invasive bacterial infections. Olaciregui et al concluded that CRP and PCT were equally strong predictors of SBI in young febrile infants, but that PCT was again more useful to detect invasive bacterial infections [37].

In an attempt to exclude the presence of SBI in young febrile infants, low-risk criteria, i.e. the so-called Rochester criteria, were proposed [39,40]. These criteria combine clinical signs and symptoms, and additional diagnostic testing results, appearing useful for safely ruling out SBI [41]. As a drawback, these low-risk criteria were based on expert opinion, rather than on evidence, and did not include CRP or PCT. Future studies looking at the scientific rationale for its predictors and the role of CRP and PCT in addition to these low-risk criteria should be encouraged. A meta-analysis showed that a PCT level ≤0.3 ng/mL was associated with a lower relative risk (RR 3.97, 95% CI 3.41–4.62) of having SBI in young febrile infants aged ≤90 days than the reported RR of the Rochester criteria (RR 30.6, 95% CI 7.0–68.13, and RR 8.75, 95% CI 2.29–15.2, for infants untreated and treated with antibiotics respectively) [41,42]. Hence, the authors concluded that a single value of PCT was inferior to the validated low-risk criteria.

Studies looking into CRP and PCT have also been performed in neonatal intensive care units, although comparative studies between CRP and PCT are lacking. A meta-analysis covering 16 studies, involving 1959 neonates, concluded that PCT was a discriminating marker for neonatal sepsis with an ROC area of 0.87; for neonates with suspected late onset sepsis (>72 hours of life) ROC area was 0.95 versus ROC area of 0.78 for early onset sepsis [43]. Numerous noninfectious reasons have been identified that contribute to a physiological rise in CRP in healthy neonates in the first 72 hours of life, limiting the value of single measurements of CRP [44]. Serial measurements of CRP were shown to be useful for guiding antibiotic treatment in neonates [45-47]. Levels of CRP <10 mg/L, taken >24 hours apart, supported the decision to safely discontinue antibiotics after 48 hours [48,49] and a decline of CRP within 4 days was a measure of treatment response [50]. Serial measurements of CRP have now been recommended by the UK's National Institute of Health and Care Excellence (NICE) clinical guidelines of managing neonatal sepsis [51]. Much the same appears to be valid for serial PCT measurements as initial studies have shown that serial measurements of PCT reduced the duration of antibiotic use [52]. Further studies on serial PCT measurements in larger cohorts of febrile neonates are currently being conducted [53].

BIOMARKERS IN CHILDREN WITH SUSPECTED APPENDICITIS

Biomarkers play an often debated role in establishing a diagnosis of appendicitis. One review (1011 suspected cases, 636 confirmed) showed that CRP was the most useful biomarker in children with suspected appendicitis (**Table 5.2**) [54]. Furthermore, PCT was found to be the most accurate biomarker in diagnosing complicated appendicitis, with a pooled sensitivity of 0.62 (95% CI 0.33–0.84), a specificity of 0.94 (95% CI 0.90–0.96) and an ROC area of 0.94 (95% CI 0.91–0.96). Correctly, the authors stress the importance of clinical findings when interpreting values of biomarkers. Another review evaluated clinical prediction rules for the detection of appendicitis in children [55]. Overall, the Pediatric Appendicitis Score (PAS) and Migration, Anorexia, Nausea/vomiting, Tenderness in the right lower quadrant, Rebound pain, Elevation in temperature, Leukocytosis, Shift (MANTRELS) to the left)/Alvarado Score were the most often and best-validated prediction models, with the PAS performing better than the MANTRELS score. However, neither was sufficiently accurate to reliably rule out appendicitis, and high-quality studies were infrequent. Also, neither CRP nor PCT was used in any of the prediction models investigated, leaving options for future research.

Table 5.2 Diagnostic performance of biomarkers in children with suspected appendicitis*					
Biomarkers	Sensitivity (95% CI)	Specificity (95% CI)	Positive LR (95% CI)	Negative LR (95% CI)	ROC-area (95%z` CI)
C-reactive protein	0.57 (0.39–0.73)	0.87 (0.58–0.97)	4.48 (1.17–17.07)	0.40 (0.26–0.63)	0.75 (0.71–0.78)
Procalcitonin	0.33 (0.21–0.47)	0.89 (0.78–0.95)	3.03 (1.82–5.05)	0.75 (0.66–0.86)	0.65 (0.61–0.69)
White blood cell count	0.62 (0.47–0.74)	0.75 (0.55–0.89)	2.50 (1.47–4.23)	0.51 (0.41–0.63)	0.72 (0.68–0.76)

*Seven studies, including both adult and paediatric populations, pooled estimates [54].
CI, confidence interval; LR, likelihood ratio; ROC, receiver operating characteristic.

BIOMARKERS IN CHILDREN AT RISK FOR SEPTIC ARTHRITIS

CRP has been acknowledged as a valuable marker in differentiating septic arthritis from transient synovitis [56-62]. Particularly in combination with fever (temperature ≥ 38.5°C), inability to weight bear, white blood cell (WBC) count 12.0×109/L, and erythrocyte sedimentation rate (ESR) ≥40 mm/h. However, studies are mostly retrospective, include small numbers, and their results have not been replicated in subsequent studies. A systematic review looking at the diagnostic value of PCT for septic arthritis, including both paediatric (two studies included) and adult studies, concluded that PCT was not useful in detecting septic arthritis but could be helpful in excluding the diagnosis [63]. The largest prospective paediatric study included 339 children of whom 8 had confirmed and 40 presumed septic arthritis. The specificity of PCT in confirmed septic arthritis at a cut-off of 0.5 ng/mL was 0.97 (95% CI 0.94–0.99), the sensitivity 0.25 (95% CI 0.30–0.65), the positive predictive value 0.18 (95% CI 0.20–0.52) and the negative predictive value 0.98 (95% CI 0.96–0.99) [64]. Only one study compared CRP and PCT in children at risk of septic arthritis [44 children of whom 12 (27%) had septic arthritis], in which PCT had higher specificities but lower sensitivities than CRP [65]. In conclusion, large prospective observational studies are lacking, in particular studies comparing CRP and PCT, but biomarkers appear useful for ruling out diagnosis of septic arthritis.

THE ROLE OF CRP AND PCT IN PREDICTING VESICOURETHRAL REFLUX AND RENAL SCARRING

PCT and CRP have been linked to predicting VUR and future renal scarring in children with pyelonephritis. A systematic review including 1011 patients (pyelonephritis in 61% and late scarring in 26%) from 18 studies showed an association between elevated levels of PCT and the presence of acute pyelonephritis and renal scarring. PCT at a cut-off level of 0.5 ng/mL had a sensitivity of 0.71 (95% CI 0.67–0.74) and a specificity of 0.72 (95% CI 0.67–0.76) for predicting acute pyelonephritis, and a sensitivity of 0.79 (95% CI 0.71–0.85) and a specificity of 0.50 (95% CI 0.45–0.54) for predicting renal scarring [66]. Likewise, a meta-analysis using data of 1280 children, of whom 199 (16%) had renal scarring, concluded CRP >40 mg/L to be an important predictor in a prediction model for renal scarring following a first UTI [67]. An additional study reported a superior diagnostic ability of PCT over CRP and WBC for predicting both acute pyelonephritis as well as the presence of renal scarring [68]. Similarly, another review, spanning 12 studies and 526 children with a first UTI, of whom 10% had VUR grade 3 or higher, concluded that PCT at a cut-off of 0.5 ng/mL was a sensitive and validated predictor for VUR grade ≥3 with a sensitivity of 0.83 (95% CI, 0.71–0.91) and a specificity of 0.43 (95% CI 0.38–0.47) [69]. Altogether, PCT and CRP appear sensitive, but no so much specific markers for renal scarring, and PCT for high-grade VUR.

BIOMARKERS IN CHILDREN WITH FEBRILE NEUTROPENIA

Children with febrile neutropenia comprise another group of patients with large diagnostic uncertainty presenting to the ED. A systematic review and meta-analysis evaluating CRP and PCT in diagnosing severe infections in children with febrile neutropenia included a total of 10 studies that assessed PCT and 8 studies looking at CRP [70]. The incidence of serious infections, and in particular bacterial sepsis, was considerably higher than those reported in the general population of febrile children, ranging from 30% (304/1031 patients) in the PCT studies to 56% (741/1316 patients) in the CRP studies. The authors concluded that PCT and CRP are valuable but by no means ideal diagnostic tests for diagnosing serious infections in this population (**Table 5.3**). Another systematic review reported on 37 studies involving 4689 episodes of febrile neutropenia in children. The authors of this review came to similar conclusions, but commented on the great heterogeneity between the studies and the paucity of reproducible findings; therefore, increasing the difficulty of pooling data and making generalisable clinical recommendations. In this study, PCT had slightly better discriminative ability than CRP [71].

OTHER BIOMARKERS IN THE DIAGNOSTIC ASSESSMENT OF FEBRILE CHILDREN

Notably, both reviews by Yo et al and van den Bruel et al concluded that PCT and CRP outperformed the traditionally often used WBC (**Table 5.2**) [10,22]. This was reiterated in a large cohort of febrile children described by De et al [72]. They found an ROC area of WBC of 0.65 (95% CI 0.63–0.68), clearly less than those reported of CRP and PCT. At the commonly used cut-off of WBC >15×109/L sensitivity was only 0.47 (95% CI 0.43–0.50) and specificity was 0.76 (95% CI 0.74–0.77), resulting in a positive LR of 1.93 (95% CI 1.75–2.13) and negative LR of 0.70 (95% CI 0.65–0.75). Many other biomarkers have been investigated, mostly in intensive care settings, in neonates or in children with increased risk of having SBI such as febrile neutropenic children. Although some markers were useful in these selected patient populations, there was no proven benefit of any of these above CRP or PCT in secondary care. Van den Bruel et al showed that ESR (one study, positive LR 2.49, negative LR 0.34), interleukine-1 (one study, positive LR 1.90, negative LR 0.46), interleukine-6 (2 studies, range positive LR 2.29–2.74, negative LR 0.33–0.50), interleukine-8 (one study, positive LR 1.89, negative LR 0.77) lacked diagnostic values and they identified a shortage of properly conducted studies [10]. Likewise, absolute neutrophil count (two studies, positive LR 1.06–1.38, negative LR 0.90–0.93), differential left shift (one study, positive LR 1.90, negative LR 0.91), granulocyte rods (three studies, range positive LR 1.45–3.05, negative LR 0.65–0.97) had limited diagnostic values.

Table 5.3. Diagnostic performance of biomarkers in children with febrile neutropenia*							
Biomarkers	No. of studies	Sensitivity (95% CI)	Specificity (95% CI)	Positive LR (95% CI)	Negative LR (95% CI)	ROC-area (95% CI)	Diagnostic Odds ratio (95% CI)
C-reactive protein	8	0.75 (0.61–0.85)	0.62 (0.49–0.73)	1.79 (1.46–2.66)	0.40 (0.26–0.63)	0.74 (0.70–0.78)	4.85 (2.58–9.12)
Procalcitonin	10	0.59 (0.42–0.74)	0.76 (0.64–0.85)	2.50 (1.64–3.81)	0.54 (0.37–0.78)	0.75 (0.71–0.78)	4.82 (2.10–11.08)

* Pooled estimates [70].
CI, confidence interval; LR, likelihood ratio; ROC, receiver operating characteristic.

DISCUSSION

Several systematic reviews show the near identical diagnostic properties of CRP and PCT in the general population of febrile children visiting the ED. In a number of observational studies PCT appeared a better marker in young febrile children, in children with short duration of fever and for detecting invasive bacterial infections such as sepsis and meningitis. It is not yet completely clear which children are benefitted from both PCT and CRP: some studies suggest that having either CRP or PCT is as beneficial as determining both biomarkers in most situations. However, the lab-score combining CRP, PCT and urinalysis has proven its value in several studies.

Differences between studies addressing prediction of SBI in febrile children hinder the interpretation and generalisability of findings [73]. For example, different cut-offs have been used to calculate and compare diagnostic performances of CRP and PCT, with only a few studies reporting diagnostic values for a range of different cut-offs. Also, there are substantial differences in target populations and differences in the reference standard for defining SBI. Another issue is that SBIs are often considered one homogeneous group, rather than a heterogeneous group of infections with distinct clinical and diagnostic characteristics. Some studies resorted to reporting on the prediction of one type of SBI, whereas others presented subgroup analysis nested within the cohort of all SBI. However, these approaches and thus failing to consider all children at risk for SBI will usually result in biased results. For a number of specific infections, evidence for the use of biomarkers is scarce and additional properly designed studies are called for. The diagnostic value of serial measurements of CRP and PCT in an emergency care setting is unclear. The effect of (serial) biomarkers on outcomes such as length of stay, hospitalisation rates and antibiotics prescribing rates needs further investigating.

CRP and PCT are useful in the diagnostic evaluation of febrile children at risk for SBI at the ED. Naturally, using biomarkers as a diagnostic tool in the evaluation of febrile children should always be supportive of a clinical impression and working diagnosis. However, some evidence suggests that routinely using biomarkers in febrile children will identify children with an SBI that would otherwise have been missed on clinical judgment only [3,74]. Conversely, high levels of CRP or PCT in a child that is clinically at subjectively low risk for SBI, should warrant a reassessment and safety netting prior to discharge home. Moreover, clinicians must balance the harms and costs of routinely testing all children with fever against the risks of missing children with SBI. SBI potentially have an aggressive clinical course with significant morbidity and mortality, and early detection of SBI in those children is needed. Deciding between PCT and CRP will depend on local preferences mainly, while considering that the scientific evidence for CRP is somewhat more extensive. Additionally, at present CRP is the cheaper of the two tests and CRP is available as a validated quantitative bedside test [10,75].

SUMMARY

Distinguishing children with serious bacterial infections from children with self-limiting febrile disease in emergency care settings can be challenging. C-reactive protein and procalcitonin have been shown to be useful diagnostic tools guiding medical decision making, both as solitary markers and combined, such as in the Lab-score, to determine SBI. Reviewing existing literature showed that CRP and PCT have equal diagnostic properties, with some evidence suggesting that PCT is more useful in young febrile infants and in children with a short duration of fever. There is clear evidence supporting the superior qualities of CRP and PCT compared with WBC count in detecting SBI. Limited evidence is available on serial measurements of CRP and PCT in paediatric emergency care for identifying children with SBI. Two studies reported a reduced duration of antibiotic treatment guided by serial PCT values, but no effect on initial prescribing rates. In children at risk of appendicitis, CRP and PCT seem to have moderate diagnostic value. CRP and PCT do appear valuable in the assessment of children at risk of septic arthritis, although comparative studies are lacking. Furthermore, PCT has potential for determining which children are at greatest risk for having dilating vesicourethral reflux (VUR) and renal scarring following a urinary tract infection. In conclusion, CRP and PCT have repeatedly been shown to be useful in the diagnostic evaluation of febrile children at risk for SBI at the emergency department, with neither outperforming the other.

Key points for clinical practice

- CRP and PCT are both equally suitable markers for ruling in or ruling out serious bacterial infections (SBIs) in children with fever.
- Cut-offs of 20 mg/L for CRP or 0.5 ng/mL for PCT are useful for ruling out SBI.
- Cut-offs of 80 mg/L for CRP or 2.0 ng/mL for PCT are useful for ruling in SBI.
- Given the high diagnostic value of biomarkers in addition to clinical signs, we recommend performing a CRP or PCT in all children with an increased risk for SBI as, for example detected by the warning signs by the guideline of NICE for the management of febrile children.
- CRP and PCT values should always be interpreted in light of the clinical context and not be used for decisive but rather as supportive tools in clinical decision making.

REFERENCES

1. Alpern ER, Stanley RM, Gorelick MH, et al. Epidemiology of a pediatric emergency medicine research network: the PECARN Core Data Project. Pediatr Emerg Care 2006; 22:689–699.
2. Hay AD, Heron J, Ness A, et al. The prevalence of symptoms and consultations in pre-school children in the Avon Longitudinal Study of Parents and Children (ALSPAC): a prospective cohort study. Fam Pract 2005; 22:367–374.
3. Craig JC, Williams GJ, Jones M, et al. The accuracy of clinical symptoms and signs for the diagnosis of serious bacterial infection in young febrile children: prospective cohort study of 15 781 febrile illnesses. BMJ 2010; 340:c1594.
4. Nijman RG, Vergouwe Y, Thompson M, et al. Clinical prediction model to aid emergency doctors managing febrile children at risk of serious bacterial infections: diagnostic study. BMJ 2013; 346:f1706.
5. Martin NG, Sadarangani M, Pollard AJ, et al. Hospital admission rates for meningitis and septicaemia caused by Haemophilus influenzae, Neisseria meningitidis, and Streptococcus pneumoniae in children in England over five decades: a population-based observational study. Lancet Infect Dis 2014; 14:397–405.
6. Crocetti M, Moghbeli N, Serwint J. Fever phobia revisited: have parental misconceptions about fever changed in 20 years? Pediatrics 2001; 107:1241–1246.
7. Gill PJ, Goldacre MJ, Mant D, et al. Increase in emergency admissions to hospital for children aged under 15 in England, 1999-2010: national database analysis. Arch Dis Child 2013; 98:328–334.
8. Thompson MJ, Ninis N, Perera R, et al. Clinical recognition of meningococcal disease in children and adolescents. Lancet 2006; 367:397–403.
9. Van den Bruel A, Haj-Hassan T, Thompson M, et al. Diagnostic value of clinical features at presentation to identify serious infection in children in developed countries: a systematic review. Lancet 2010; 375:834–845.

10. Van den Bruel A, Thompson MJ, Haj-Hassan T, et al. Diagnostic value of laboratory tests in identifying serious infections in febrile children: systematic review. BMJ 2011; 342:d3082.
11. Oostenbrink R, Nijman RG, Venmans L, et al. Richtlijn: koorts in de tweede lijn bij kinderen 0-16 jaar. Nederlandse Vereniging voor Kindergeneeskunde (Dutch Society of Paediatrics). Utrecht: NVK, 2014.
12. Galetto-Lacour A, Zamora SA, Andreola B, et al. Validation of a laboratory risk index score for the identification of severe bacterial infection in children with fever without source. Arch Dis Child 2010; 95:968–973.
13. Mallett S, Halligan S, Thompson M, et al. Interpreting diagnostic accuracy studies for patient care. BMJ 2012; 345:e3999.
14. Tillett WS, Francis T. Serological reactions in pneumonia with a non-protein somatic fraction of pneumococcus. J Exp Med 1930; 52:561–571.
15. Assicot M, Gendrel D, Carsin H, et al. High serum procalcitonin concentrations in patients with sepsis and infection. Lancet 1993; 341:515–518.
16. Becker KL, Nylen ES, White JC, et al. Clinical review 167: procalcitonin and the calcitonin gene family of peptides in inflammation, infection, and sepsis: a journey from calcitonin back to its precursors. J Clin Endocrinol Metab 2004; 89:1512–1525.
17. Pierce R, Bigham MT, Giuliano JS Jr. Use of procalcitonin for the prediction and treatment of acute bacterial infection in children. Curr Opin Pediatr 2014; 26:292–298.
18. Luaces-Cubells C, Mintegi S, Garcia-Garcia JJ, et al. Procalcitonin to detect invasive bacterial infection in non-toxic-appearing infants with fever without apparent source in the emergency department. Pediatr Infect Dis J 2012; 31:645–647.
19. Pratt A, Attia MW. Duration of fever and markers of serious bacterial infection in young febrile children. Pediatr Int 2007; 49:31–35.
20. Andreola B, Bressan S, Callegaro S, et al. Procalcitonin and C-reactive protein as diagnostic markers of severe bacterial infections in febrile infants and children in the emergency department. Pediatr Infect Dis J 2007; 26:672–677.
21. Sanders S, Barnett A, Correa-Velez I, et al. Systematic review of the diagnostic accuracy of C-reactive protein to detect bacterial infection in nonhospitalized infants and children with fever. J Pediatr 2008; 153:570–574.
22. Yo CH, Hsieh PS, Lee SH, et al. Comparison of the test characteristics of procalcitonin to C-reactive protein and leukocytosis for the detection of serious bacterial infections in children presenting with fever without source: a systematic review and meta-analysis. Ann Emerg Med 2012; 60:591–600.
23. Lacour AG, Gervaix A, Zamora SA, et al. Procalcitonin, IL-6, IL-8, IL-1 receptor antagonist and C-reactive protein as identificators of serious bacterial infections in children with fever without localising signs. Eur J Pediatr 2001; 160:95–100.
24. Galetto-Lacour A, Zamora SA, Gervaix A. Bedside procalcitonin and C-reactive protein tests in children with fever without localizing signs of infection seen in a referral center. Pediatrics 2003; 112:1054–1060.
25. Thayyil S, Shenoy M, Hamaluba M, et al. Is procalcitonin useful in early diagnosis of serious bacterial infections in children? Acta Paediatr 2005; 94:155–158.
26. Lacour AG, Zamora SA, Gervaix A. A score identifying serious bacterial infections in children with fever without source. Pediatr Infect Dis J 2008; 27:654–656.
27. Bressan S, Gomez B, Mintegi S, et al. Diagnostic performance of the lab-score in predicting severe and invasive bacterial infections in well-appearing young febrile infants. Pediatr Infect Dis J 2012; 31:1239–1244.
28. Nijman RG, Moll HA, Smit FJ, et al. C-reactive protein, procalcitonin and the lab-score for detecting serious bacterial infections in febrile children at the emergency department: a prospective observational study.. Pediatr Infect Dis J 2014; 33:e273–e279.
29. Lacroix L, Manzano S, Vandertuin L, et al. Impact of the lab-score on antibiotic prescription rate in children with fever without source: a randomized controlled trial.. PLoS One. 2014; 9:e115061.
30. Flood RG, Badik J, Aronoff SC. The utility of serum C-reactive protein in differentiating bacterial from nonbacterial pneumonia in children: a meta-analysis of 1230 children. Pediatr Infect Dis J 2008; 27:95–99.
31. Harris H, Clark J, Coote N, et al. British Thoracic Society guidelines for the management of community acquired pneumonia in children: update 2011. Thorax 2011; 66:ii1–ii23.
32. Oostenbrink R, Thompson M, Lakhanpaul M, et al. Children with fever and cough at emergency care: diagnostic accuracy of a clinical model to identify children at low risk of pneumonia. Eur J Emerg Med 2012; 20:273–280.

33. Segal I, Ehrlichman M, Urbach J, et al. Use of time from fever onset improves the diagnostic accuracy of C-reactive protein in identifying bacterial infections. Arch Dis Child 2014; 99:974–978.

34. Baer G, Baumann P, Buettcher M, et al. Procalcitonin guidance to reduce antibiotic treatment of lower respiratory tract infection in children and adolescents (ProPAED): a randomized controlled trial. PLoS One 2013; 8:e68419.

35. Manzano S, Bailey B, Girodias JB, et al. Impact of procalcitonin on the management of children aged 1 to 36 months presenting with fever without source: a randomized controlled trial. Am J Emerg Med 2010; 28:647–653.

36. Schuetz P, Muller B, Christ-Crain M, et al. Procalcitonin to initiate or discontinue antibiotics in acute respiratory tract infections. Cochrane Database Syst Rev 2012; 9:CD007498.

37. Olaciregui I, Hernandez U, Munoz JA, et al. Markers that predict serious bacterial infection in infants under 3 months of age presenting with fever of unknown origin. Arch Dis Child 2009; 94:501–505.

38. Gomez B, Bressan S, Mintegi S, et al. Diagnostic value of procalcitonin in well-appearing young febrile infants. Pediatrics 2012; 130:815–822.

39. Dagan R, Powell KR, Hall CB, et al. Identification of infants unlikely to have serious bacterial infection although hospitalized for suspected sepsis. J Pediatr 1985; 107:855–860.

40. Anbar RD, Richardson-de Corral V, O'Malley PJ. Difficulties in universal application of criteria identifying infants at low risk for serious bacterial infection. J Pediatr 1986; 109:483–485.

41. Huppler AR, Eickhoff JC, Wald ER. Performance of low-risk criteria in the evaluation of young infants with fever: review of the literature. Pediatrics 2010; 125:228–233.

42. England JT, Del Vecchio MT, Aronoff SC. Use of serum procalcitonin in evaluation of febrile infants: a meta-analysis of 2317 patients. J Emerg Med 2014; 47:682–688.

43. Vouloumanou EK, Plessa E, Karageorgopoulos DE, et al. Serum procalcitonin as a diagnostic marker for neonatal sepsis: a systematic review and meta-analysis. Intensive Care Med 2011; 37:747–762.

44. Hofer N, Zacharias E, Muller W, et al. An update on the use of C-reactive protein in early-onset neonatal sepsis: current insights and new tasks. Neonatology 2012; 102:25–36.

45. Ehl S, Gering B, Bartmann P, et al. C-reactive protein is a useful marker for guiding duration of antibiotic therapy in suspected neonatal bacterial infection. Pediatrics 1997; 99:216–221.

46. Bomela HN, Ballot DE, Cory BJ, et al. Use of C-reactive protein to guide duration of empiric antibiotic therapy in suspected early neonatal sepsis. Pediatr Infect Dis J 2000; 19:531–535.

47. Philip AG, Mills PC. Use of C-reactive protein in minimizing antibiotic exposure: experience with infants initially admitted to a well-baby nursery. Pediatrics 2000; 106:E4.

48. Hengst JM. The role of C-reactive protein in the evaluation and management of infants with suspected sepsis. Adv Neonatal Care 2003; 3:3–13.

49. Benitz WE, Han MY, Madan A, et al. Serial serum C-reactive protein levels in the diagnosis of neonatal infection. Pediatrics 1998; 102:E41.

50. Ronnestad A, Abrahamsen TG, Gaustad P, et al. C-reactive protein (CRP) response patterns in neonatal septicaemia. APMIS 1999; 107:593–600.

51. National Institute of Health and Care Excellence (NICE). Clinical guideline 149: Antibiotics for the prevention and treatment of early-onset neonatal infection. London: NICE, 2012.

52. Stocker M, Fontana M, El Helou S, et al. Use of procalcitonin-guided decision-making to shorten antibiotic therapy in suspected neonatal early-onset sepsis: prospective randomized intervention trial. Neonatology 2010; 97:165–174.

53. Stocker M, Hop WC, van Rossum AM. Neonatal Procalcitonin Intervention Study (NeoPInS): Effect of Procalcitonin-guided decision making on duration of antibiotic therapy in suspected neonatal early-onset sepsis: A multi-centre randomized superiority and non-inferiority Intervention Study. BMC Pediatr 2010; 10:89.

54. Yu CW, Juan LI, Wu MH, et al. Systematic review and meta-analysis of the diagnostic accuracy of procalcitonin, C-reactive protein and white blood cell count for suspected acute appendicitis. Br J Surg 2013; 100:322–329.

55. Kulik DM, Uleryk EM, Maguire JL. Does this child have appendicitis? A systematic review of clinical prediction rules for children with acute abdominal pain. J Clin Epidemiol 2013; 66:95–104.

56. Kocher MS, Zurakowski D, Kasser JR. Differentiating between septic arthritis and transient synovitis of the hip in children: an evidence-based clinical prediction algorithm. J Bone Joint Surg Am 1999; 81:1662–1670.

57. Jung ST, Rowe SM, Moon ES, et al. Significance of laboratory and radiologic findings for differentiating between septic arthritis and transient synovitis of the hip. J Pediatr Orthop 2003; 23:368–372.

58. Caird MS, Flynn JM, Leung YL, et al. Factors distinguishing septic arthritis from transient synovitis of the hip in children. A prospective study. J Bone Joint Surg Am 2006; 88:1251–1257.

59. Kocher MS, Mandiga R, Zurakowski D, et al. Validation of a clinical prediction rule for the differentiation between septic arthritis and transient synovitis of the hip in children. J Bone Joint Surg Am 2004; 86-A:1629–1635.

60. Luhmann SJ, Jones A, Schootman M, et al. Differentiation between septic arthritis and transient synovitis of the hip in children with clinical prediction algorithms. J Bone Joint Surg Am 2004; 86-A:956–962.

61. Sultan J, Hughes PJ. Septic arthritis or transient synovitis of the hip in children: the value of clinical prediction algorithms. J Bone Joint Surg Br 2010; 92:1289–1293.

62. Singhal R, Perry DC, Khan FN, et al. The use of CRP within a clinical prediction algorithm for the differentiation of septic arthritis and transient synovitis in children. J Bone Joint Surg Br 2011; 93:1556–1561.

63. Shen CJ, Wu MS, Lin KH, et al. The use of procalcitonin in the diagnosis of bone and joint infection: a systemic review and meta-analysis. Eur J Clin Microbiol Infect Dis 2013; 32:807–814.

64. Faesch S, Cojocaru B, Hennequin C, et al. Can procalcitonin measurement help the diagnosis of osteomyelitis and septic arthritis? A prospective trial. Ital J Pediatr 2009; 35:33.

65. Butbul-Aviel Y, Koren A, Halevy R, et al. Procalcitonin as a diagnostic aid in osteomyelitis and septic arthritis. Pediatr Emerg Care 2005; 21:828–832.

66. Leroy S, Fernandez-Lopez A, Nikfar R, et al. Association of procalcitonin with acute pyelonephritis and renal scars in pediatric UTI. Pediatrics 2013; 131:870–879.

67. Shaikh N, Craig JC, Rovers MM, et al. Identification of children and adolescents at risk for renal scarring after a first urinary tract infection: a meta-analysis with individual patient data. JAMA Pediatr 2014; 168:893–900.

68. Sheu JN, Chang HM, Chen SM, et al. The role of procalcitonin for acute pyelonephritis and subsequent renal scarring in infants and young children. J Urol 2011; 186:2002–2008.

69. Leroy S, Romanello C, Galetto-Lacour A, et al. Procalcitonin is a predictor for high-grade vesicoureteral reflux in children: meta-analysis of individual patient data. J Pediatr 2011; 159:644–651, e644.

70. Lin SG, Hou TY, Huang DH, et al. Role of procalcitonin in the diagnosis of severe infection in pediatric patients with fever and Neutropenia – a systemic review and meta-analysis. Pediatr Infect Dis J 2012; 31:e182–e188.

71. Haeusler GM, Carlesse F, Phillips RS. An updated systematic review and meta-analysis of the predictive value of serum biomarkers in the assessment of fever during neutropenia in children with cancer. Pediatr Infect Dis J 2013; 32:e390–e396.

72. De S, Williams GJ, Hayen A, et al. Value of white cell count in predicting serious bacterial infection in febrile children under 5 years of age. Arch Dis Child 2014; 99:493–499.

73. Oostenbrink R, Thompson M, Steyerberg EW. Barriers to translating diagnostic research in febrile children to clinical practice: a systematic review. Arch Dis Child 2012; 97:667–672.

74. Mintegi S, Benito J, Astobiza E, et al. Well appearing young infants with fever without known source in the emergency department: are lumbar punctures always necessary? Eur J Emerg Med 2010; 17:167–169.

75. Monteny M, ten Brinke MH, van Brakel J, et al. Point-of-care C-reactive protein testing in febrile children in general practice. Clin Chem Lab Med 2006; 44:1428–1432.

Chapter 6

Respiratory syncytial virus prophylaxis in congenital heart disease

Robert MR Tulloh, Jessica Green

INTRODUCTION

Respiratory syncytial virus infection is a common and serious infection in the first year of life, especially in those with critical congenital heart disease (CHD). Preventative methods for this illness have not been identified and children still die each year from severe pneumonia, or have their operations cancelled.

We discuss the various options and controversies surrounding this subject in order to highlight the difficulties in managing such an important group of patients.

RESPIRATORY SYNCYTIAL VIRUS INFECTION

Respiratory syncytial virus (RSV) is a common cause of lower respiratory tract infections in young children and infants. Most children (over 80%) will acquire an infection before the age of 2, with bronchiolitis and pneumonia being the most prevalent manifestations. Within this group of children, the ones who acquire the most severe infections and in the high-risk category are those with an underlying condition, such as CHD. The seriousness of an underlying condition was illustrated in a UK cohort study carried out from 1999 to 2007 which found that the 8.6% of children who died in the intensive care unit with RSV infection had a comorbidity [1]. In addition, the UK Office of Population and Census Surveys showed that over 30% of those children who die with RSV infection have CHD [2].

The fatality rates of children born with CHD who acquire RSV infection ranged between 2% and 37%, whereas the rates for children with no underlying condition were consistently below 1% [3]. In addition, RSV appears to cause myocarditis with a resultant low cardiac output [4] which is clearly a poor prognostic indicator for children with CHD, and even more in the perioperative period. Owing to the higher risk of death among children with CHD, there needs to be an effective method of prevention of RSV for these patients. If RSV is present on a cardiac unit, it can significantly affect the running of the department, causing delay in surgery by 6 weeks, or leading to significant postoperative complications [5,6].

Robert MR Tulloh DM FRCPCH, Department of Congenital Heart Disease, Bristol Royal Hospital for Children, Bristol, UK. Email Robert.Tulloh@Bristol.ac.uk (for correspondence)

Jessica Green, Department of Congenital Heart Disease, Bristol Royal Hospital for Children, Bristol, UK

At present, there is inconsistency in the interpretation of the current guidelines as well as controversy about the best protocol to protect children with CHD against RSV [7]. In addition, although therapy and prophylaxis exist, cost and overall effectiveness remain an issue.

CURRENT THERAPIES AGAINST ACTIVE RSV INFECTION

Ribavirin is used as a therapy to prevent the replication of ribonucleic acid (RNA) and deoxyribonucleic acid. It is usually administered in an aerosol form and is currently the only US Food and Drug Administration (US FDA) approved antiviral treatment for RSV. There appears to be evidence for its efficacy in very acute patients with a severe infection and children in need of a lung transplant [8,9].

However, the cost is high and the aerosol method of delivery is not easy to administer. Furthermore, the potential danger to staff administering the drug means that its use has to be limited and it is, therefore, less effective.

There is also a lack of sufficient, comparable evidence for ribavirin efficacy in an RSV infection. Many studies conducted have not included children with significant comorbidities, such as CHD. Furthermore, one study that used nebulised water as a placebo found that the water might have, in fact, had a damaging effect on pulmonary function [10]. Therefore, despite its FDA approval, the American College of Paediatrics does not favour the use of ribavirin in the treatment of RSV infection [8].

Other forms of treatment

There have been a number of drugs trialled to treat RSV infections such as corticosteroids, nebulised adrenaline and bronchodilators. Among these, the corticosteroids and bronchodilators appear to have some use in treating symptoms of bronchiolitis in the short term, but do not reduce the length of hospitalisation. Corticosteroids, especially, do not appear to reduce the long-term complications like asthma or wheezing. As such, there has been no clinical evidence that these treatments should be recommended to infants with acute bronchiolitis [11].

EMERGING THERAPY

Cathelicidins are host defence proteins that are integral parts of the immune system. The human cathelicidin, LL-37, has been shown to reduce cell apoptosis in RSV-infected cells and decreases the vulnerability of bronchial epithelial cells to infection [8]. When used alongside vitamin D, the expression of LL-37 increases. This supplementation may be used in the future for development of a new and beneficial peptide treatment although safety studies need to be performed. Vitamin D may have value as a relatively cost-effective therapy that could be used as a complementary treatment [8].

Antisense anti-RSV drugs act by targeting mRNA and viral RNA oligonucleotides, inhibiting protein synthesis [12]. It is true that these drugs still need to be tested for their efficacy in a large trial for infants, but so far, results have shown potential [12].

On balance, there is a need for a prophylactic treatment that is effective in children with CHD while also being cost effective.

PROPHYLAXIS WITH PALIVIZUMAB

Palivizumab, a passive monoclonal antibody, is the only recommended prophylaxis for preterm-born infants with CHD or immune deficiency. It is available as an intramuscular injectable form, which is administered to children and infants five times during the RSV infection season. It appears to be safe, with few adverse incidents.

The main study of the drug, which demonstrated efficacy, showed a reduction in the severity of illness and in children with haemodynamically significant heart disease showed reductions in hospitalisations for RSV infections [13]. The study demonstrated that the prophylaxis was safe, and this was important given the previous uncertainties with the intravenous form of the therapy, monoclonal antibody (RespiGam), which had appeared to cause increased cyanotic episodes in children with CHD [14]. It was heavily stratified by cardiac morphology and physiology, allowing clinicians to conclude that there was no added risk to children with cyanotic CHD. The study was worldwide and included 1287 children between 1998 and 2002 with haemodynamically significant CHD (hsCHD). With palivizumab, a 45% reduction in hospitalisations was seen and it was most effective in children below 6 months of age. There was a significant reduction in the number of infants in whom oxygen therapy was required.

As a result of this study, drug and medicine agencies (FDA and European Medicines Agency) approved palivizumab for use in children with CHD, in addition to those with prematurity and chronic lung disease. A series of guidelines were produced which allowed the clinician to decide on the suitability of prophylaxis in different countries. The American Academy of Paediatrics (updated) [15], the British Paediatric Cardiac Association (**Table 6.1**) [16], in addition to the German, the Canadian and the French organisations, present individual guidelines relevant to the country of origin. These were mostly harmonised and in agreement to the benefits of palivizumab. They have been updated in the United States to include more preterm babies who have been shown to benefit from the reduction in RSV infection severity.

After the production of these guidelines, most countries in the world took up palivizumab as the best means of protecting high-risk patients. The number of hospitalisations of children with CHD in California in the 'pre-palivizumab era' in 2000–2002 was compared to that in the 'post-palivizumab era' from 2004 to 2006 [17]. The total number of hospitalisations decreased by 22% in the post-palivizumab era, giving a total saving of $897,864. Some of the reduction was due to the improvement in clinical practice in these years. It was also noted [17] that the effectiveness of palivizumab was more

Table 6.1 Summary of BPCA guidelines for prophylaxis with Palivizumab in CHD 2005		
Recommended*	**Exclude**	**Consider**
Documented hsCHD	Uncomplicated CHD such as ASD or small VSD	Older infants 1–2 years depending on CHD
Pulmonary hypertension		Case by case consideration
Partially corrected hsCHD		
Expected admission to hospital during RSV season		
* Some of these recommendations extend beyond the current licence. ASD, atrial septal defect; CHD, congenital heart disease; hsCHD, haemodynamically significant congenital heart disease; RSV, respiratory syncytial virus; VSD, ventricular septal defect.		

remarkable when clinical trials were conducted in a controlled study environment, rather than the results of the real-life hospitalisations in California. This was credited to increased patient and health care worker adherence and overall compliance during the clinical trials, which is described as being 'artificially elevated'.

Administration of palivizumab

Palivizumab is administered as a 15 mg/kg intramuscular injection, once a month for 5 months, over the course of the RSV season, which is from about November to March [18]. There are a few problems with its cost effectiveness [19]. Firstly, it simply costs more to administer five doses of a drug rather than one or two. The cost of a 50 mg vial of palivizumab is $725.

The preparation is only available as a single 50 mg or 100 mg vial, although many health care workers share one vial among patients to save on cost. Care is needed to administer the injections within 6–12 hours of vial entry, as the preparation does not contain preservatives [18].

In addition, there is the cost of each injection visit, not just for the health care provision but also for the patient's travel and potential time off work for the parents or guardian. The American Hospital Directory states that it costs $70 on average for an injection visit [20]. These variables among others, such as cost of an average RSV hospitalisation and quality of life with or without palivizumab, were used by Elhassan et al [19] to determine the cost effectiveness of palivizumab with the current method of treatment. They concluded that palivizumab was not a cost-effective treatment and the present guidelines for prophylaxis should be reviewed [19]. Furthermore, it takes significant organisation to administer injections. The children have their weights recorded 3 days before their appointment, and each child has a dedicated nurse seeing them on the same day every month [18].

Health care economics

There is an ongoing debate as to whether palivizumab is cost effective and this seems to be the main reason of limiting prophylaxis to a high-risk group of children.

A Canadian study found that it costs $8292 (Canadian) more to treat a patient with palivizumab than to give hospital treatment. Despite this, there was a 42% drop in hospital admissions in children below the age of 2 after it was introduced [28]. The incremental cost-effectiveness ratio has been shown to be €13,849 in a Spanish study [29], which is considerably lower than the European cut-off for a new drug of €30,000. However, in the United Kingdom repeated attempts have been made to demonstrate cost-effectiveness and these have not been successful, except in the group of very preterm babies and in those who are born preterm and who have CHD [30]. An American study showed that the cost of life per year saved was approximately $100,000 in children with hsCHD and that the total cost to the US economy would be $20m for 5000 patients [31] Clearly, this needs to be thought through, and unless the cost–benefit equation can be shifted, then prophylaxis with palivizumab will be difficult to justify on a cost basis alone.

Current guidelines

As a result of these uncertainties, over efficacy and cost effectiveness, new guidelines have been produced by the American Academy of Paediatrics (**Table 6.2**) [15].

Table 6.2 Patients who should receive palivizumab prophylaxis, according to current AAP* guidelines (2014)
Infants born at 28 weeks' gestation or earlier
Infants born at <32 weeks' gestation who require supplemental oxygen >28 days
Infants and children <2 years old who are severely immunocompromised
Infants with hsCHD[†]
Infants with pulmonary abnormalities or neuromuscular disease
*American Academy of Pediatrics [†]hsCHD, haemodynamically significant congenital heart disease.

There is further uncertainty in other countries too, some not recommending RSV prophylaxis with palivizumab at all. In the United Kingdom, the Joint Committee on Vaccination and Immunization has advised that it is cost effective only in preterm babies or those with immune deficiency. Infants and older children with hsCHD are to be given palivizumab prophylaxis if they are also born preterm. However, there is also flexibility to include those with any condition in which the clinician feels that there is a risk to the patient and a benefit to be gained from prophylaxis. As a result, some clinicians are adhering to the BPCA (now BCCA) guidelines, some have their own guidelines; some are protecting the highest risk patients – those with severe pulmonary hypertension or very delicately balanced circulations, such as those with hypoplastic left heart syndrome and the Norwood operation [32]. Also, it is common practice to give prophylaxis to those infants who are resident on the intensive care unit over the winter months in order to protect those high risk patients, e.g. with pulmonary hypertension and with chronic lung disease.

Other controversies

One of the drawbacks of palivizumab coming to market is that many of the active projects previously in progress to discover new vaccines, antibodies and antivirals became inactive [33]. Many companies cancelled their development of new RSV drugs because they did not see RSV as a priority any more. Although it is argued that RSV kills more patients than acquired immune deficient syndrome (AIDS) in many parts of the world, AIDS still receive a much higher proportion of the research and development budget than RSV.

MOTAVIZUMAB

This has enhanced affinity for the RSV F glycoprotein, the same viral target used by palivizumab [21]. About 6635 preterm infants with chronic lung disease of prematurity were entered into a study of motavizumab against palivizumab. Both had similar low rates of hospitalisation for RSV but there was a 50% relative reduction in outpatient, RSV-specific, medically attended lower respiratory tract infection with motavizumab [22].

Similarly, when used in a comparison with palivizumab in children with hsCHD, the results for efficacy were promising, with a similar reduction in the severity of illness. However, owing to the lack of improved prevention of hospitalisation with motavizumab and an increased occurrence of skin rash reaction in this group, the US FDA have not approved it, and the manufacturer has decided not to pursue licensing at this time.

PREVENTION OF SPREAD

Following guidelines for hand washing and adhering to hygiene standards are well known elements of preventing infection spread. As RSV can survive for up to 7 hours on surfaces [23], it can easily be spread to other patients, especially if these patients have a comorbidity such as CHD. Indeed, hygiene education is a vitally important aspect of health care, and it has been proposed that parents should be informed of these controls during the antenatal stay and before they are discharged [18]. Risk factors for spread of RSV infection also include sibling contact, nursery school contacts, parental smoking and Down's syndrome (with narrow upper airways). Reducing the risk of transmission of RSV infection has had a major impact in both family and hospital environments.

CHRONIC WHEEZING

RSV infection has been implicated in the genesis of wheezing in the first few years of life. An observational, prospective study of children born after 35 weeks' gestation or less found that those who had received palivizumab had a much lower occurrence of wheezing later on when compared with those children who had not been given the prophylaxis [24,25]. In addition, it has been shown that children undergoing cardiac surgery are more likely to have respiratory complications than controls if they have suffered from RSV infection prior to operation, which can also be mistaken for heart failure [5].

OTHER RISK FACTORS

Down's syndrome increases the risk of contracting severe RSV infection, especially in the presence of hsCHD [26]. It is suggested that the close proximity to other children and carers, in addition to the smaller airways in this population, enhances the risk of severe disease. Many countries will add this group to their list of infants to be included in a prophylaxis programme. It is also clear that those infants who are born at later gestations also have an equal or even greater risk of infection, especially in the presence of hsCHD [27].

VACCINES

A live vaccine would relieve much of the burden from RSV patients in hospitals [18] and, if the safety were proven, would be a far more cost-effective treatment than the five monthly injections needed with palivizumab. It would not only reduce the acute effects of the RSV infection but also the long-term implications such as viral wheeze [25].

However, there have been some barriers to the research of a new vaccine. The search for a candidate for an effective vaccine is still ongoing. The formalin-inactivated F1-vaccine, trialled in the 1960s, enhanced the severity of the infection [34]. Therefore, the search is on for a safe and effective, live attenuated vaccine. Medi-534 is a live attenuated, intranasal vaccine that has been found to be useful against RSV. It had good results when used on adults in the early stages of trials, and even proved to be a safe treatment for children [34]. However, Medi-534 has thus far been a fairly weak vaccine, being 'minimally immunogenic'.

A drawback of using live vaccines is that high-risk children who might benefit the most from a vaccine may have a weaker, more susceptible immune system with an unpredictable response.

CONCLUSION

With RSV being one of the leading causes of lower respiratory tract infections in infants, it is imperative that there is effective prevention. RSV can result in severe infection in high-risk children, sometimes leading to death. Palivizumab is the only approved treatment, and studies have proved its success. However, it is relatively expensive and had not yet been found to be a cost-effective treatment. There is a plethora of guidelines, leading to confusion as to the best course of action.

THE FUTURE

We, look forward to the development of effective protection against RSV, especially for our most vulnerable population. We have concentrated on those with hsCHD in this chapter, but there are several populations at risk, with prematurity, immune deficiency and old-age chronic lung disease being among them.

Key points for clinical practice

- RSV is a serious and frequent infection in young children with comorbidities such as CHD.
- Up to 30% of those children dying with RSV infection have CHD.
- Palivizumab is the only recognised prophylaxis against RSV infection and is recommended in certain patient groups (**Table 6.2**).
- There is no current effective treatment for RSV infection.
- There is still controversy surrounding the best groups of children to be protected and the cost effectiveness of palivizumab.
- An effective vaccine is not yet available for RSV infection.

REFERENCES

1. Thorburn K. Pre-existing disease is associated with a significantly higher risk of death in severe respiratory syncytial virus infection. Arch Dis Child 2009; 94:99–103.
2. HMSO. Office of Population Censuses and Surveys. Mortality statistics: childhood, infant and perinatal, England and Wales (Series DH3) No.34. London: Office for National Statistics, 2001.
3. Welliver RC Sr, Checchia PA, Bauman JH, et al. Fatality rates in published reports of RSV hospitalizations among high-risk and otherwise healthy children. Curr Med Res Opin. 2010; 26:2175–2181.
4. Caplow J, McBride SC, Steil GM, et al. Changes in cardiac output and stroke volume as measured by non-invasive CO monitoring in infants with RSV bronchiolitis. J Clin Monit Comput. 2012; 26:197–205.
5. Tulloh R, Flanders L. Does RSV infection cause increased morbidity and pulmonary hypertension in children with Congenital Heart Disease undergoing cardiac surgery? Arch Dis Child 2011;96:Suppl 1 A37-A38 doi:10.1136/adc.2011.212563.80.
6. Khongphatthanayothin A, Wong PC, Samara Y, et al. Impact of respiratory syncytial virus infection on surgery for congenital heart disease: postoperative course and outcome. Crit Care Med 1999; 27:1974–1981.
7. Tulloh RM, Bury S. Prevention and prophylaxis of respiratory syncytial virus in pediatric cardiology: a UK perspective. Future Cardiol 2014; 10:235–242.
8. Turner TL, Kopp BT, Paul G, et al. Respiratory syncytial virus: current and emerging treatment options. Clinicoecon Outcome.
9. Pelaez A, Lyon GM, Force SD, et al. Efficacy of oral ribavirin in lung transplant patients with respiratory syncytial virus lower respiratory tract infection. J Heart Lung Transplant 2009; 28:67–71.

10. Moler FW, Bandy KP, Custer JR. Ribavirin therapy for acute bronchiolitis: need for appropriate controls. J Pediatr 1991; 119:509–510.
11. Scottish Intercollegiate Guidelines Network (SIGN). Bronchiolitis: a national clinical guideline, 2006. Edinburgh: SIGN, 2006.
12. Empey KM, Peebles RS Jr, Kolls JK. Pharmacologic advances in the treatment and prevention of respiratory syncytial virus. Clin Infect Dis 2010;50:1258–1267.
13. Feltes TF, Cabalka AK, Meissner HC, et al. Palivizumab prophylaxis reduces hospitalization due to respiratory syncytial virus in young children with hemodynamically significant congenital heart disease. J Pediatr 2003;143:532–540.
14. Groothuis JR, Simoes EA, Hemming VG. Respiratory syncytial virus (RSV) infection in preterm infants and the protective effects of RSV immune globulin (RSVIG). Respiratory Syncytial Virus Immune Globulin Study Group. Pediatrics 1995; 95:463–467.
15. American Academy of Pediatrics Committee on Infectious D, American Academy of Pediatrics Bronchiolitis Guidelines C. Updated guidance for palivizumab prophylaxis among infants and young children at increased risk of hospitalization for respiratory syncytial virus infection. Pediatrics 2014; 134:415–420.
16. Tulloh R, Marsh M, Blackburn M, et al. Recommendations for the use of palivizumab as prophylaxis against respiratory syncytial virus in infants with congenital cardiac disease. Cardiology Young 2003; 13:420–423.
17. Chang RK, Chen AY. Impact of palivizumab on RSV hospitalizations for children with hemodynamically significant congenital heart disease. Pediatr Cardiol 2010; 31:90–95. PubMed PMID: 19915892. Pubmed
18. Paes BA, Mitchell I, Banerji A, et al. A decade of respiratory syncytial virus epidemiology and prophylaxis: translating evidence into everyday clinical practice. Can Respir J 2011; 18:e10–e09.
19. Elhassan NO, Sorbero ME, Hall CB, et al. Cost-effectiveness analysis of palivizumab in premature infants without chronic lung disease. Arch Pediatr Adolesc Med 2006; 160:1070–1076.
20. American Hospital Directory. 2004–2015 Cost Report Data Resources, LLC. Louisville: American-Hospital Directory Inc., 2015.
21. Wu H, Pfarr DS, Johnson S, Development of motavizuab, an ultra-potent antibody for the prevention of respiratory syncytial virus infection in the upper and lower respiratory tract. J Mol Biol 2007; 368:652–665.
22. Feltes TF, Sondheimer HM, Tulloh RM, et al. A randomized controlled trial of motavizumab versus palivizumab for the prophylaxis of serious respiratory syncytial virus disease in children with hemodynamically significant congenital heart disease. Pediatr Res 2011; 70:186–191.
23. Hall CB, Douglas RG Jr, Geiman JM. Possible transmission by fomites of respiratory syncytial virus. J Infect Dis 1980; 141:98–102.
24. Antibody against RSV helps prevent wheeze in infants. BMJ 2013; 346:f3089.
25. Yoshihara S, Kusuda S, Mochizuki H, et al. Effect of palivizumab prophylaxis on subsequent recurrent wheezing in preterm infants. Pediatrics 2013; 132:811–818.
26. Paes B, Mitchell I, Yi H, et al. Hospitalization for respiratory syncytial virus illness in Down syndrome following prophylaxis with palivizumab. Pediatr Infect Dis J Pediatr Infect Dis J 2014; 33:e29–33.
27. Carbonell-Estrany X, Simoes EA, Fullarton JR, et al. Validation of a model to predict hospitalization due to RSV of infants born at 33–35 weeks' gestation. J Perinat Med 2010; 38:411–417.
28. Harris KC, Anis AH, Crosby MC, et al. Economic evaluation of palivizumab in children with congenital heart disease: a Canadian perspective. Can J Cardiol 2011; 27:523, e11–15.
29. Nuijten MJ, Wittenberg W. Cost effectiveness of palivizumab in Spain: an analysis using observational data. Eur J Health Econ 2010; 11:105–15. PubMed PMID: 19967425.
30. Nuijten MJ, Wittenberg W, Lebmeier M. Cost effectiveness of palivizumab for respiratory syncytial virus prophylaxis in high-risk children: a UK analysis. PharmacoEconomics 2007; 25:55–71.
31. Yount LE, Mahle WT. Economic analysis of palivizumab in infants with congenital heart disease. Pediatrics 2004; 114:1606–1611.
32. Tulloh RM, Feltes TF. The European Forum for Clinical Management: prophylaxis against the respiratory syncytial virus in infants and young children with congenital cardiac disease. Cardiol Young. 2005; 15:274–278.
33. Maggon K, Barik S. New drugs and treatment for respiratory syncytial virus. Rev Med Virol. 2004; 14:149–168.
34. Gomez M, Mufson MA, Dubovsky F, et al. Phase-I study MEDI-534, of a live, attenuated intranasal vaccine against respiratory syncytial virus and parainfluenza-3 virus in seropositive children. Pediatr Infect Dis J. 2009; 28:655–658.

Chapter 7

Noninvasive measurements of airway inflammation in children

Louise Fleming, Prasad Nagakumar

INTRODUCTION

Asthma is a chronic inflammatory disease characterised by reversible variable airflow obstruction. It manifests as recurrent episodes of wheeze, breathlessness, cough and chest tightness [1]. It is the most common chronic paediatric disease in the United Kingdom where the prevalence of childhood asthma is one of the highest in Europe [2]. The majority of children with asthma are well controlled on intermittent bronchodilators or a low dose of inhaled corticosteroids (ICS). However, despite the fact that asthma is common and effective treatments are available, it is not always straightforward to manage. There is no gold standard for the diagnosis of asthma; a significant minority of children require high-intensity treatment and have significant morbidity including poor school attendance and high health care costs [3]; finally, there is no standardised way to monitor treatment response and disease progression. Airway inflammation is not only a key pathological process in asthma but also an important therapeutic target. The development of tests for the noninvasive measurement of airway inflammation affords the opportunity to measure inflammation in the clinical setting. This chapter will review the noninvasive measures of airway inflammation most commonly used in clinical practice and examine their utility in the diagnosis and monitoring of asthma. We will also briefly discuss tests used in the research setting and describe potential future developments.

PATHOPHYSIOLOGY – AIRWAY INFLAMMATION

The key pathological mechanisms underlying asthma are inflammation, airway remodelling and airway hyper-responsiveness (AHR) which lead to the clinical manifestations of asthma [4]. Airway inflammation is a consistent finding in asthma but the type and severity of the inflammation can be variable and can be absent if anti-inflammatory treatment, principally ICS, is effective. Many cell types and mediators play an important role in the inflammatory process in asthma. Inflammation in the airways

Louise Fleming MBChB MD MRCPCH, National Heart and Lung Institute, Imperial College, London, UK. Email: l.fleming@rbht.nhs.uk (for correspondence)

Prasad Nagakumar MBBS MRCPCH, Respiratory Paediatrics, Royal Brompton and Harefield NHS Foundation Trust, UK is characterised by the presence of mast cells, eosinophils, neutrophils, T lymphocytes and dendritic cells. These cells produce >100 known inflammatory mediators. Asthma is traditionally thought to be a disease driven by the adaptive immune system via T-helper 2 (Th2) cells. The Th2 cytokines interleukin-4 (IL-4), IL5 and IL-13 are thought to play an important role in the induction and pathogenesis of asthma and orchestrate eosinophilic inflammation. IL-4 induces the production of immunoglobulin E (IgE) by B cells; IL-5 is crucial for activation of eosinophils and their migration into the lung and IL-13 is associated with AHR, mucus hypersecretion and airway remodelling [5]. However, it has been shown that children with severe therapy-resistant asthma have evidence of airway remodelling and eosinophilic inflammation in the absence of the classical Th2 cytokines (IL-4, IL-5 and IL-13) suggesting that other mediators are driving this process [6].

Lower airway sampling performed during bronchoscopy, including bronchoalveolar lavage and endobronchial biopsy can provide information about the presence of inflammatory cells and mediators in the airway lumen and within the airway wall. These methods have greatly enhanced our knowledge of the underlying pathophysiology of asthma. In the individual patient, these invasive measures of inflammation enable detailed inflammatory characterisation. However, they provide only a snapshot taken at a single time point. In adults, these samples can be collected relatively easily as flexible bronchoscopy is performed under light sedation; however, even then very frequent sampling is not possible and bronchoscopy can only be performed in the specialist setting. There are even greater limitations in paediatric practice: bronchoscopy is carried out under general anaesthesia; bronchoscopy is only carried out if clinically indicated and is rarely repeated; and it would be unethical to carry out bronchoscopy in a child purely for research. In view of these limitations, identification of biological molecules (biomarkers) from a noninvasive source such as sputum, exhaled breath or urine is crucial and can help us to further our understanding as well as the management of asthma. The most commonly used methods for measuring inflammatory biomarkers are induced sputum and exhaled nitric oxide (FeNO), although other measurements in exhaled breath are a fertile area of research. An ideal biomarker would be one that aids diagnosis, gives an indication of current control and changes in which it would indicate therapeutic efficacy and risk of future complications. Furthermore, any such marker should be easily measurable at regular intervals with minimal inconvenience to the patient. **Table 7.1** summarises the invasive and noninvasive tests useful in childhood asthma.

Table 7.1 Summary of invasive and noninvasive tests of inflammation in childhood asthma	
Invasive	**Noninvasive**
Flexible bronchoscopy Bronchoalveolar lavage Bronchial biopsy Bronchial brushings Blood investigations	Direct measures of airway inflammation: • Induced sputum • Exhaled nitric oxide • Exhaled breath condensate Indirect measures of airway inflammation: • Urinary metabolites • Salivary metabolites

NONINVASIVE MARKERS OF AIRWAY INFLAMMATION

Direct measures of airway inflammation

Induced sputum

The presence of catarrh or phlegm as a characteristic of asthma features in some of the earliest writings on this disease. In Maimondes' 12th century 'Treatise on Asthma', he describes a patient who 'gasps for air until phlegm is expelled' and recommends chicken soup to expectorate the phlegm [7]. Paul Ehlrich first described the eosinophil in 1879 and shortly afterwards blood eosinophils were reported as being important in asthma [8]. Reports of examining sputum in asthmatic patients and treatment guided by the cellular composition were published over 50 years ago [9].

Sputum induction is considered the gold standard for noninvasively measuring airway inflammation. Analysis of airway inflammatory cells in induced sputum provides information regarding the cellular composition of the airway lumen. Induced cells reflect bronchoalveolar lavage, bronchial washings and, to a lesser extent, bronchial biopsy findings in children with asthma [10]. Mucus production is often increased in asthmatics however; it can be difficult for asthmatics to expectorate spontaneously, particularly when well. A method for inducing sputum in adult asthmatics was first described by Pin et al in 1993 [11]. The patient inhales nebulised hypertonic saline (3.5-4.5%) for a specified time (usually for 15–20 minutes). It has been shown to be safe, even for children with severe asthma [12]. Hypertonic saline triggers sputum production by various mechanisms including activation of mast cells and nerve endings, initiating cough, changes in airway surface liquid and improved mucociliary clearance [13]. The principal readout is the differential inflammatory cell count, usually expressed as a percentage of 400 nonsquamous cells on a stained cytospin preparation (**Figure 7.1**), although the total cell

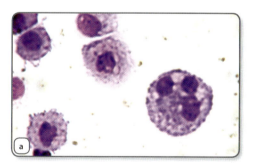

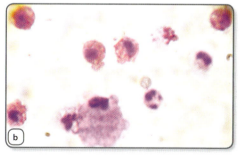

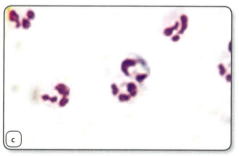

Figure 7.1 Stained cytospins. (a) Normal sputum sample comprised predominantly of macrophages. (b) Predominantly eosinophilic sample (eosinophils are stained red). (c) Predominantly neutrophilc sputum sample.

count can also be reported. Numerous inflammatory mediators can be measured in the fluid phase of sputum (supernatant). These include cytokines, chemokines and proteases.

Sputum induction allows longitudinal assessment of airway inflammation and a large number of patients can be studied. However, it is not widely available in clinical practice: it is time consuming, requires expertise and appropriate laboratory facilities to process the sputum. It can cause unwanted effects such as cough and bronchoconstriction and the taste is unpleasant. However, it is generally well tolerated and sputum induction is successful in 70–90%, with success increasing with age.

Based on cellularity in induced sputum, asthma can be classified into the following phenotypes: eosinophilic (high eosinophils), neutrophilic (high neutrophils), mixed cellular (high eosoinophils and neutrophils) and paucigranulocytic (low eosinophils and neutrophils) [20]. The reported cut-points for high eosinophils and neutrophils are variable depending on the population studied, but, in general, an eosinophil level of >2.5% and a neutrophil level of >54% are used to define sputum eosinophilic and neutrophilic phenotypes in children.

This classification of asthma based on airway inflammation has clinical implications as it reflects the underlying pathology. The presence of eosinophils is characteristic of many, but not all, patients with asthma. Eosinophils contain inflammatory enzymes, generate leukotrienes and express a wide variety of proinflammatory cytokines [14].

Neutrophils can also be present in increased numbers in the airways of asthmatics, particularly during an exacerbation and in the presence of smoking, although the precise role of neutrophils in asthma is not known. Neutrophils are recruited into the airway mainly by IL-8. It has been suggested that adults with a predominantly neutrophilic infiltrate represent a distinct subgroup of asthma with a different pathogenesis to those with predominantly eosinophilic inflammation [15–19]. However, this is not the case in children where airway neutrophila is highly variable and not a stable phenotype [20]. In children, significant neutrophilia in sputum or bronchoalveolar lavage usully reflects presence of an infection.

Clinical utility of induced sputum in asthmatics

Sputum cellularity reflects the pathology in proximal airways. Although identifying the presence of eosinophils in sputum provides complimentary information to the other physiological measures, the role of sputum induction in routine clinical practice to monitor children with asthma has not yet been established. Sputum phenotypes are not stable over time [20], and there is variability in the quantity and quality of sputum obtained longitudinally.

Diagnosis

Current diagnosis of asthma is largely based on symptoms and measures of lung function. A number of studies have demonstrated that sputum eosinophils are significantly higher in children with asthma than healthy controls [21,22]. However, a study in steroid naïve children whose asthma was diagnosed on the basis of symptoms and positive methacholine challenge or bronchodilator responsiveness found that 36% had no evidence of sputum eosinophilia at diagnosis [23]. The conclusions which we can draw from this are somewhat limited as no studies in children have compared the validity of sputum eosinophils compared to conventional tests such as peak flow variability, spirometry, bronchodilator reversibility and AHR. One study on adults suggested that only methacholine challenge had better sensitivity and specificity than sputum eosinophils for diagnosing asthma [24]. The difficulty with such studies is the lack of a gold standard test for the diagnosis of asthma.

Assessment of steroid responsiveness

Morrow–Brown first showed that eosinophils are a predictor of steroid response over 50 years ago [9]. There is convincing evidence from a number of adult studies that eosinophils fall in response to steroids and one paediatric study has demonstrated a fall in sputum eosinophils in newly diagnosed asthmatics after 6 months of treatment with budesonide [25]. One small study of 17 children with severe asthma already treated with high-dose ICS or oral steroids demonstrated a significant fall in sputum eosinophils after intramuscular triamcinolone; however, there were similar forced expiratory volume in 1 second (FEV_1) and clinical improvements in those without sputum eosinophilia at baseline [26].

Monitoring asthma

Measurement of sputum eosinophils has been successfully incorporated into management algorithms in a number of adult studies leading to a significant reduction in exacerbations in those managed according to sputum eosinophils rather than symptoms [27-29]. Only one study in children with severe asthma has tested this strategy [30]. Although tailoring treatment based on 3 monthly sputum eosinophil counts in children did show a reduction in the exacerbation rate during the month after each visit, there was no overall difference in exacerbation rates between the symptom and sputum management groups. This may, in part, be due to the variability of inflammatory phenotype in children with asthma [20]. Interestingly, a posthoc analysis showed that there was a benefit in boys if an inflammation-based management strategy was used. Currently, there are insufficient data to state definitively what role sputum eosinophils should play in monitoring children with asthma. It is likely that certain subgroups may benefit from this strategy.

CURRENT GUIDELINES AND FUTURE DIRECTIONS

The British Thoracic Society (BTS) and Scottish Intercollegiate Guidelines Network (SIGN) guidelines recommend that for patients with difficult asthma monitoring induced sputum eosinophil counts to guide steroid treatment should be considered [31]. Although not stated explicitly, this recommendation appears to relate to adults rather than children. They also suggest that measures of eosinophilic airway inflammation are closely linked to a positive response to corticosteroids (CS). However, there is no specific recommendation.

A recent study in adults has shown eosinophil peroxidise assay is a reliable surrogate marker of eosinophils [32]. This is promising, particularly, as it can help us to avoid the labour-intensive processing currently needed to quantify sputum eosinophils. However, the study needs to be replicated in a large cohort before it is available for routine clinical care. In paediatrics, sputum induction remains a research tool, although we use it in our clinic as part of the assessment of steroid response.

FRACTIONAL EXHALED NITRIC OXIDE (FENO)

Studies in 1980s showed that nitric oxide plays an important role as a biological messenger. It was first detected in exhaled breath in 1991. Two years later, Alving et al identified, for the first time, elevated levels of fractional exhaled nitric oxide (FeNO) in adult asthmatics [33]. Nelson et al showed similar results in children with asthma in 1997 [34].

Nitric oxide synthases (NOS) are key enzymes in the biosynthesis of NO. Three isoforms of these enzymes exist; endothelial and neuronal NOS, which are constitutively active and inducible NO (iNOS). iNOS generates nitric oxide in the lungs by oxidation of L-arginine and is induced by proinflammatory cytokines within airway epithelial cells. A wide variety of cells in the airways including epithelial cells, endothelial cells, nerves and inflammatory cells produce nitric oxide [35]. Proinflammatory cytokines which activate iNOS are also involved in the eosinophilic inflammatory response. A high concentration of nitric oxide in airways is attributed to eosinophilic inflammation; however, it should be noted that FeNO is an indirect measure as only small amounts of NO are produced by eosinophils.

Clinical utility of FeNO

In the clinical setting, FeNO can be easily measured with the help of variety of commercially available devices. Guidelines recommend that FeNO is measured online at a steady flow rate of 50 mL/s [36]. It fulfils many of the criteria for the ideal biomarker: it is easy to measure; reproducible; a result is available almost immediately; there is no discomfort to the patient and newer; more portable devices mean that it can be measured in a variety of settings, including primary care and the home. However, the clinical utility of FeNO remains contentious.

Diagnosis

Recent guidelines have suggested clinically important cut-points for FeNO. The American Thoracic Society (ATS) suggests that low FeNO (<25 ppb or <20 ppb in children <12 years) indicates that eosinophilic inflammation and responsiveness to CS are less likely and that high FeNO (>50 ppb or >35 ppb in children <12 years) indicates a high likelihood of steroid responsive eosinophilic inflammation [36]. However, there is a complex relationship between FeNO and atopy and elevated levels of FeNO are frequently seen in atopic children, independent of asthma [37]. Furthermore, discordance between levels of sputum eosinophils and FeNO is a common finding in childhood asthma and there is an inconsistent relationship between sputum eosinophils and FeNO in the individual [38A]. The National Institute for Clinical Excellence (NICE) recommends that FeNO can help to diagnose asthma in combination with other diagnostic tests in those with an intermediate probability of asthma [38B].

Assessment of steroid response

Numerous studies in adults and children have demonstrated that FeNO levels can be lowered by treatment with CS. It is likely that CS reduce FeNO by a direct effect on transcription of iNOS and indirectly by reduction in the levels of stimulatory inflammatory cytokines. This observation has led to the incorporation of FeNO as a measure of adherence. McNicholl et al used directly observed therapy (DOT) in adults with poorly controlled asthma and high levels of FeNO [39]. Those whose FeNO levels fell rapidly once DOT was initiated were found to have poor prescription uptake of ICS. This has also been our finding in our severe asthma cohort admitted for further investigations. FeNO levels frequently fall following initiation of supervised administration of inhaled steroids along with improved symptom score and reduction of asthma exacerbations.

Monitoring asthma

The results of studies incorporating FeNO into management strategies have been largely disappointing [40–43]. One recent study in children achieved a reduction in exacerbations at the expense of a significantly higher ICS dose [44]. At present, the evidence is lacking to support the widespread use of FeNO to guide management in clinical practice [45].

Exhaled breath condensate (EBC)

This is collected by cooling or freezing exhaled air. Several inflammatory mediators of inflammation including cytokines (IL-6, IL-8, tumour necrosis factor), hydrogen peroxide, peptides, leukotrienes and EBC pH have been studied. The composition of EBC is thought to reflect airway-lining fluid and concentrations of a number of these mediators have been shown to be relate to underlying airway inflammation. Low pH in EBC is said to indicate airway inflammation and, therefore, represents poor asthma control [46]. A meta-analysis of eight studies measuring hydrogen peroxide levels in EBC showed that these levels were increased in patients with asthma and may be a useful biomarker [47]. However, the subgroup analysis of the only two paediatric studies included in the meta-analysis did not show statistical difference between children with asthma and healthy controls. Associations have also been found between other mediators such as 8 isoprostanes and cysteinyl leukotriene, and measures of airway obstruction and asthma control. However, most mediators are present in very low concentrations, can be difficult to measure and no reference values are available. It is unlikely that a single biomarker from EBC will be useful in the clinical setting.

More recently, there have been some promising data from patterns of volatile organic compounds (VOCs) measured in exhaled breath, using an 'electronic nose'. The breath is collected during tidal breathing into nalophan bags. The gas can be analysed by a number of platforms including mass spectrometry, which produce metabolomic fingerprints. This has been shown to discriminate the exhaled breath of asthmatics from healthy controls [48]. In a study of children with asthma and preschool wheeze, the unbiased clustering of VOC patterns produced distinct clinical clusters suggesting that metabolomics in exhaled air may be useful for phenotyping childhood asthma [49].

CLINICAL IMPLICATIONS

EBC remains as a research tool and clinical application of metabolomic fingerprints is some way off. It is anticipated that in the future these fingerprints will be translated into a more clinically meaningful readout reflecting the likelihood of a diagnosis of asthma or asthma phanotype.

INDIRECT MEASURES OF AIRWAY INFLAMMATION

Urine metabolites

Urine is rich in metabolites and it can be easily obtained from children of any age. Urinary leukotriene E4 (LTE4) levels reflect systemic cysteinyl leukotriene production which is increased during an exacerbation, particularly related to viral infections. It has been shown that asthmatic children with a higher LTE4/FeNO ratio respond better to montelukast (leukotriene antagonist) over ICS [50]. Bromotyrosine, a marker of eosinophil activation, has been shown to track asthma control and predict future risk of an exacerbation in asthmatic children [51]. In a study of 135 children, nuclear magnetic resonance (NMR) spectroscopy was used to measure 70 metabolites in urine and correctly diagnosed asthma in 94% of the cases [52]. NMR technology is promising as large numbers of metabolites can be quantified without significant pretreatment of the sample. Urine analysis of 623 Norwegian children found elevated levels of urinary phthalates and a modest association with asthma control. Exposure to phthalates can occur via a variety of routes including indoor air particulate matter. Whether this is a clinically useful measure remains to be seen.

CLINICAL IMPLICATIONS

There are only a small number of clinical studies which have used urinary metabolites to diagnose asthma, predict exacerbations and treatment outcomes. Furthermore, the variable and often very short half life of these metabolites, and need for sophisticated equipment for analysing samples preclude their use in routine practice at present.

SALIVARY METABOLITES

Recently, there is a growing interest in the analysis of inflammatory markers in saliva. A study by Little et al has shown that using Principle Component Analysis, a strong correlation was noted between symptom control and salivary levels of eotaxin, IL-5, IL-8 in children and adults with asthma [53]. Salivary eosinophilic cationic protein and other proteomics were also investigated as possible salivary biomarkers. Further studies are needed to assess clinical utility.

CONCLUSION

Asthma is a heterogeneous disease. Inflammation is a key pathological process across all phenotypes although patterns of inflammation and clinical manifestations can be variable. Noninvasive measurement of inflammation in the clinical setting affords the opportunity to improve diagnosis, management and monitoring of asthma in children. Each biomarker discussed in this chapter has advantages and disadvantages and it is unlikely that a single noninvasive biomarker of inflammation will provide all the answers. Patterns of biomarkers used in combination with symptoms and physiology will likely have the greatest clinical utility. The explosion in 'omics' technologies and refinement of analytical and knowledge management platforms have the potential to identify biomarkers which will introduce a step change in the identification of clinically meaningful phenotypes that can be used to develop individualised targeted treatment plans [54]. The outcome of one such study in adults and children with asthma that has taken an unbiased approach to the integration of large-omics data sets is eagerly awaited [55]. In the meantime, sputum eosinophils and FeNO remain the most commonly used measures of inflammation in clinical practice. They clearly have a role to play, particularly, in specialist centres and in children with more severe asthma. However, while they provide an important piece of the asthma puzzle, they do not provide the whole answer.

Key points for clinical practice

- Asthma is a heterogeneous airway inflammatory disease diagnosed clinically with no gold standard test available for diagnosis.
- Noninvasive measures of airway inflammation complement physiological measurements and have the potential to improve paediatric asthma management and guide treatment.
- Noninvasive markers of inflammation help us to identify clinically meaningful phenotypes.
- FeNO and induced sputum analysis are currently the most frequently available markers for airway inflammation.
- Further research, particularly, in standardising protocols for analysis of saliva and urine for inflammatory biomarkers in asthma is necessary before they are available for routine clinical care.

REFERENCES

1. Bousquet J, Mantzouranis E, Cruz AA, et al. Uniform definition of asthma severity, control, and exacerbations: document presented for the World Health Organization Consultation on Severe Asthma. J Allergy Clin Immunol 2010; 126:926–938.
2. Asher MI, Montefort S, Bjorksten B, et al. Worldwide time trends in the prevalence of symptoms of asthma, allergic rhinoconjunctivitis, and eczema in childhood: ISAAC Phases One and Three repeat multicountry cross-sectional surveys. Lancet 2006; 368:733–743.
3. Bush A, Saglani S. Management of severe asthma in children. Lancet 2010; 376:814–825.
4. Busse WW, Lemanske RF Jr. Asthma. N Engl J Med 2001; 344:350–362.
5. Doherty T, Broide D. Cytokines and growth factors in airway remodeling in asthma. Curr Opin Immunol 2007; 19:676–680.
6. Bossley CJ, Fleming L, Gupta A, et al. Pediatric severe asthma is characterized by eosinophilia and remodeling without T(H)2 cytokines. J Allergy Clin Immunol 2012; 129:974–982.
7. Rosner F. Moses maimonides and diseases of the chest. Chest 1971; 60:68–72.
8. Venge P. Eosinophils and respiratory disease. Respir Med 2001; 95:168–169.
9. Morrow Brown H. Treatment of chronic asthma with prednisolone significance of eosinophils in the sputum. Lancet 1958; 272:1245–1247.
10. Lex C, Ferreira F, Zacharasiewicz A, et al. Airway eosinophilia in children with severe asthma: predictive values of noninvasive tests. Am J Respir Crit Care Med 2006; 174:1286–1291.
11. Pin I, Gibson PG, Kolendowicz R, et al. Use of induced sputum cell counts to investigate airway inflammation in asthma. Thorax 1992; 47:25–29.
12. Lex C, Payne DN, Zacharasiewicz A, et al. Sputum induction in children with difficult asthma: safety, feasibility, and inflammatory cell pattern. Pediatr Pulmonol 2005; 39:318–324.
13. Gould NS, Gauthier S, Kariya CT, et al. Hypertonic saline increases lung epithelial lining fluid glutathione and thiocyanate: two protective CFTR-dependent thiols against oxidative injury. Respir Res 2010; 11:119.
14. Rothenberg ME, Hogan SP. The eosinophil. Annu Rev Immunol 2006; 24:147–174.
15. Gibson PG, Simpson JL, Saltos N. Heterogeneity of airway inflammation in persistent asthma: evidence of neutrophilic inflammation and increased sputum interleukin-8. Chest 2001; 119:1329–1336.
16. Green RH, Brightling CE, Woltmann G, et al. Analysis of induced sputum in adults with asthma: identification of subgroup with isolated sputum neutrophilia and poor response to inhaled corticosteroids. Thorax 2002; 57:875–879.
17. Jatakanon A, Uasuf C, Maziak W, et al. Neutrophilic inflammation in severe persistent asthma. Am J Respir Crit Care Med 1999; 160:1532–1539.
18. Shaw DE, Berry MA, Hargadon B, et al. Association between neutrophilic airway inflammation and airflow limitation in adults with asthma. Chest 2007; 132:1871–1875.
19. Simpson JL, Grissell TV, Douwes J, et al. Innate immune activation in neutrophilic asthma and bronchiectasis. Thorax 2007; 62:211–218.

20. Fleming L, Tsartsali L, Wilson N, et al. Sputum inflammatory phenotypes are not stable in children with asthma. Thorax 2012; 67:675–681.
21. Gibson PG, Simpson JL, Chalmers AC, et al. Airway eosinophilia is associated with wheeze but is uncommon in children with persistent cough and frequent chest colds. Am J Respir Crit Care Med 2001; 164:977–981.
22. Gibson PG, Simpson JL, Hankin R, et al. Relationship between induced sputum eosinophils and the clinical pattern of childhood asthma. Thorax 2003; 58:116–121.
23. Lee YJ, Kim KW, Choi BS, et al. Clinical characteristics of eosinophilic and noneosinophilic asthma in children. Acta Paediatr 2013; 102:53–57.
24. Goldstein MF, Veza BA, Dunsky EH, et al. Comparisons of peak diurnal expiratory flow variation, postbronchodilator FEV(1) responses, and methacholine inhalation challenges in the evaluation of suspected asthma. Chest 2001; 119:1001–1010.
25. Rytila P, Pelkonen AS, Metso T, et al. Induced sputum in children with newly diagnosed mild asthma: the effect of 6 months of treatment with budesonide or disodium cromoglycate. Allergy 2004; 59:839–844.
26. Lex C, Jenkins G, Wilson NM, et al. Does sputum eosinophilia predict the response to systemic corticosteroids in children with difficult asthma? Pediatr Pulmonol 2007; 42:298–303.
27. Chlumsky J, Striz I, Terl M, et al. Strategy aimed at reduction of sputum eosinophils decreases exacerbation rate in patients with asthma. J Int Med Res 2006; 34:129–139.
28. Green RH, Brightling CE, McKenna S, et al. Asthma exacerbations and sputum eosinophil counts: a randomised controlled trial. Lancet 2002; 360:1715–1721.
29. Jayaram L, Pizzichini MM, Cook RJ, et al. Determining asthma treatment by monitoring sputum cell counts: effect on exacerbations. Eur Respir J 2006; 27:483–494.
30. Fleming L, Wilson N, Regamey N, et al. The use of non-invasive markers of inflammation to guide management in children with severe asthma. Am J Respir Crit Care Med 2009; 179:A1305.
31. British Guideline on the Management of Asthma. British Thoracic Society; Scottish Intercollegiate Guidelines Network. Thorax 2014; 69:i1–i192.
32. Nair P, Ochkur SI, Protheroe C, et al. Eosinophil peroxidase in sputum represents a unique biomarker of airway eosinophilia. Allergy 2013; 68:1177–1184.
33. Alving K, Weitzberg E, Lundberg JM. Increased amount of nitric oxide in exhaled air of asthmatics. Eur Respir J 1993; 6:1368–1370.
34. Nelson BV, Sears S, Woods J, et al. Expired nitric oxide as a marker for childhood asthma. J Pediatr 1997; 130:423–427.
35. Ricciardolo FL. cNOS-iNOS paradigm and arginase in asthma. Trends Pharmacol Sci 2003; 24:560–561.
36. Dweik RA, Boggs PB, Erzurum SC, et al. An official ATS clinical practice guideline: interpretation of exhaled nitric oxide levels (FENO) for clinical applications. Am J Respir Crit Care Med 2011; 184:602–615.
37. Franklin PJ, Turner SW, Le Souef PN, et al. Exhaled nitric oxide and asthma: complex interactions between atopy, airway responsiveness, and symptoms in a community population of children. Thorax 2003; 58:1048–1052.
38A. Fleming L, Tsartsali L, Wilson N, et al. Longitudinal relationship between sputum eosinophils and exhaled nitric oxide in children with asthma. Am J Respir Crit Care Med 2013; 188:400–402.
38B. National Institute of Health and CAre Excellence (NICE). Measuring fractional exhaled nitric oxide concentration in asthma:: NIOX MINO, NIOX VERO and NObreath. Diagnostic guidance (DG12). London; NICE, 2014.
39. McNicholl DM, Stevenson M, McGarvey LP, et al. The utility of fractional exhaled nitric oxide suppression in the identification of nonadherence in difficult asthma. Am J Respir Crit Care Med 2012; 186:1102–1108.
40. De Jongste JC, Carraro S, Hop WC, et al. Daily telemonitoring of exhaled nitric oxide and symptoms in the treatment of childhood asthma. Am J Respir Crit Care Med 2009; 179:93–97.
41. Fritsch M, Uxa S, Horak F Jr, et al. Exhaled nitric oxide in the management of childhood asthma: a prospective 6-months study. Pediatr Pulmonol 2006; 41:855–862.
42. Pijnenburg MW, Bakker EM, Hop WC, et al. Titrating steroids on exhaled nitric oxide in children with asthma: a randomized controlled trial. Am J Respir Crit Care Med 2005; 172:831–836.
43. Szefler SJ, Mitchell H, Sorkness CA, et al. Management of asthma based on exhaled nitric oxide in addition to guideline-based treatment for inner-city adolescents and young adults: a randomised controlled trial. Lancet 2008; 372:1065–1072.
44. Petsky HL, Li AM, Au CT, et al. Management based on exhaled nitric oxide levels adjusted for atopy reduces asthma exacerbations in children: A dual centre randomized controlled trial. Pediatr Pulmonol 2015 Jun;5096):535-43.

45. Petsky HL, Cates CJ, Lasserson TJ, et al. A systematic review and meta-analysis: tailoring asthma treatment on eosinophilic markers (exhaled nitric oxide or sputum eosinophils). Thorax 2012; 67:199–208.

46. Kostikas K, Papaioannou AI, Tanou K, et al. Exhaled NO and exhaled breath condensate pH in the evaluation of asthma control. Respir Med 2011; 105:526–532.

47. Teng Y, Sun P, Zhang J, et al. Hydrogen peroxide in exhaled breath condensate in patients with asthma: a promising biomarker? Chest 2011; 140:108–116.

48. Montuschi P, Santonico M, Mondino C, et al. Diagnostic performance of an electronic nose, fractional exhaled nitric oxide, and lung function testing in asthma. Chest 2010; 137:790–796.

49. Brinkman P, Hashimoto S, Fleming L, et al. Unbiased clustering of children with asthma or pre-school wheeze using the U-BIOPRED electronic nose platform. Eur Res Soc Congrs, 2015.

50. Rabinovitch N. Urinary leukotriene E4. Immunol Allergy Clin North Am 2007; 27:651–664.

51. Wedes SH, Wu W, Comhair SA, et al. Urinary bromotyrosine measures asthma control and predicts asthma exacerbations in children. J Pediatr 2011; 159:248–255.

52. Saude EJ, Skappak CD, Regush S, et al. Metabolomic profiling of asthma: diagnostic utility of urine nuclear magnetic resonance spectroscopy. J Allergy Clin Immunol 2011; 127:757–764.

53. Little FF, Delgado DM, Wexler PJ, et al. Salivary inflammatory mediator profiling and correlation to clinical disease markers in asthma. PLoS One 2014; 9:e84449.

54. Sittka A, Vera J, Lai X, et al. Asthma phenotyping, therapy, and prevention: what can we learn from systems biology? Pediatr Res 2013; 73:543–552.

55. Wheelock CE, Goss VM, Balgoma D, et al. Application of 'omics' technologies to biomarker discovery in inflammatory lung diseases. Eur Respir J 2013; 42:802–825.

Chapter 8

Advances in paediatric intensive care

Benedict T Griffiths, Shane M Tibby

INTRODUCTION

The last two decades have witnessed increasing survival rates for children admitted to the paediatric intensive care unit (PICU), despite treating a growing number of patients with complex comorbidities [1]. This has been temporally associated with major changes in two aspects of care: restructuring of intensive care provision, and better evaluation of novel and established therapies.

Changes in intensive care provision have been widespread, and include the following:

1. Improved early recognition and treatment of the at-risk and decompensating child, via mandating resuscitation courses within general paediatric training, and establishment of PICU outreach teams
2. Delivery of intensive care before and after physical PICU admission, through dedicated retrieval teams and increasing use of advanced therapies (e.g. noninvasive ventilation) outside of the PICU environment
3. Publication of PICU standards of care
4. Workforce issues, such as establishing an intercollegiate PICU curriculum for medics in the United Kingdom, and development of the advanced nurse practitioner role
5. Public health initiatives, e.g. successful vaccination programmes for a range of infectious organisms, such as meningococcus and pneumococcus.

The second area, therapeutic evaluation, has largely 'come of age' in the last decade. We are better at trial design and delivery, aided by a broader group of stakeholders. Research priorities and study design are now informed by national and international organisations; both generic (National Institute of Health Research bodies, such as the Medicines for Children Research Network) and speciality based (United Kingdom Paediatric Intensive Care Society Clinical Study Group). End users (i.e. parents and children) are increasingly consulted formally with respect to trial design and delivery; this is now mandatory for many grant-giving bodies. Industry engagement has improved vastly across paediatrics, aided by European and UK legislation. Research questions are more focussed (aided by standardised taxonomy for clinical syndromes, such as sepsis and acute respiratory distress syndrome

Benedict T Griffiths MBBS, Paediatric Intensive Care Unit, Evelina Children's Hospital, London, UK

Shane M Tibby MBChB, Paediatric Intensive Care Unit, Evelina Children's Hospital, London, UK. Email: shane.tibby@gstt.nhs.uk (for correspondence)

(ARDS)). The requirement for large, multicentre randomised controlled trials (RCTs) is now a given: we have recently completed two large, publically funded RCTs in the United Kingdom, each recruiting approximately 1500 patients (the two largest of their kind in the world to date). The need for facilitating meta-analysis is considered increasingly at trial design stage. In addition, there is a growing acknowledgement of transferrable knowledge from our sister intensive care unit specialties: neonatal and adult. Many therapies are now evaluated across the entire age spectrum, recent examples being therapeutic hypothermia (TH) and tight glucose control (discussed later in this chapter).

This chapter will highlight therapeutic changes in PICU care within several key areas over the last decade. As such, it is by no means an exhaustive literature review, but rather aims to highlight the interaction between organisational aspects, therapeutic evaluation and relevant studies from neonatal and adult intensive care unit that have resulted in changes in PICU care.

SEPSIS MANAGEMENT AND THE RISE OF THE CARE BUNDLE

Historically, much of the treatment for sepsis was nonstandardised and based on low-grade evidence, resulting in the formation of the International Sepsis Forum in 1999. This small group of adult health care professionals produced an evidence-based guideline in 2001, which provided the impetus for establishing the Surviving Sepsis Campaign in 2002. This international campaign comprised a much larger, expert group, resulting in the Surviving Sepsis Guidelines in 2004, with revisions in 2008 and 2012 [2]; all included paediatric-specific considerations. These guidelines were developed along the same evidence-based principles, and resulted in grading of evidence and recommendations for 15 specific aspects of sepsis, including diagnosis, initial resuscitation targets, antibiotic therapy, fluids, vasoactive agents, steroids and source control, which taken together represent the concept of a 'care bundle'. A key principle is that all aspects of a care bundle should be administered in a timely fashion, and should be deliverable across a spectrum of health care settings. The surviving sepsis guidelines were (and remain) largely consistent with the main international paediatric resuscitation guidelines and courses [Advanced Paediatric Life Support (APLS), European Pediatric Life Support (EPLS), and Paediatric Advanced Life Support (PALS)], with a cornerstone being early recognition followed by large-volume fluid resuscitation, timely antibiotic administration and, where necessary, early use of mechanical ventilation and inotropes. Surviving sepsis is now a major global initiative, and is supported by the World Federation of Pediatric Intensive and Critical Care Societies (http://www.wfpiccs.org/projects/sepsis-initiative/).

A key paper supporting and perhaps refining the sepsis care bundle concept emerged from Rivers et al in 2001 [3], which first coined the term 'early goal-directed therapy' (EGDT), and subsequently became the highest cited intensive care unit paper to date (3903 citations on Web of Science, 18 November 2014). This emergency department-based RCT utilised early resuscitation in 263 adult patients with severe sepsis and/or septic shock, targeted to physiological endpoints: for the control group, these were mean arterial pressure, central venous pressure and urine output. The treatment group (dubbed EGDT) targeted the same endpoints, with the addition of central venous oxygen saturation measurement (aiming for >70%). The hypothesis stated that central venous hypoxia represented occult, ongoing shock, which if corrected early (<6 hours after presentation, and before intensive care unit admission), would improve survival. The trial found a significantly lower mortality in the group receiving EGDT (30.5% versus 46.5%). Interestingly, both groups received similar fluid resuscitation, ventilation and inotrope use over the first 72 hours after presentation, with the key difference being that the EGDT group received the majority of these therapies early, i.e. within the first 6 hours.

Despite its landmark status, many authors highlighted weaknesses in, and unanswered questions from, the Rivers study. This led to the near simultaneous execution of three large adult RCTs across three continents over 5 years, each addressing a slightly different aspect of EGDT, but harmonised to facilitate meta-analysis. At the time of writing, all trials have been completed (>4000 patients recruited in total), two have been published fully [4,5], with results of the third being expected shortly. Of note, there were no differences in mortality between the EGDT and control groups: all were of the order of 18–20% [4,5].

The results of these studies are intriguing [4,5]: one consistent finding of note is the consistently lower mortality in the control arms (i.e. a relative reduction of >50%) compared to Rivers' and earlier studies [3]. This has led many to conclude that, rather than EGDT being noneffective, it does not add benefit when a sepsis bundle is adhered to, as seen in the control arms. For example, in both PROtocolized Care for Early Septic Shock (ProCESS) and Australasian Resuscitation in Sepsis Evaluation (ARISE) trials [4,5], all groups received on average >2 L of fluid, and >75% received antibiotics prior to randomisation (fulfilling two key aspects of the 3-hour Surviving Sepsis Campaign bundle) [2]. It may be that, provided we get the basics right in terms of accurate clinical assessment and regular review, the more advanced aspects of EGDT (central venous oxygen saturation titration and perhaps even citing arterial lines) may be necessary for a selected group of 'nonresponding' or high-risk patients only.

Paediatric-specific evidence

Paediatric studies evaluating sepsis treatment are rare; many are low grade (e.g. cohort studies), others possess methodological limitations, and some have produced negative findings. Several high-quality RCTs have been undertaken in the developing world, whose transferability to the developed world has been limited by the diseases studied (e.g. dengue), comorbidities in the study populations, and a lack of intensive care backup.

Timing of resuscitation

The only paediatric evidence is from retrospective cohort studies; however, these have shown an apparent survival benefit when the PALS guidelines are instituted early and adhered to [6].

Early goal-directed therapy

To date, one RCT [7] has been published in Brazil (2008), comparing resuscitation based upon PALS guidelines to EGDT. The trial was halted after an interim analysis of 102 patients showed a higher 28-day mortality in the control group (39% versus 12%), which represents an extremely large effect size. Unfortunately, this trial has major methodological limitations, which question its validity and generalisability. (1) Baseline observations were not typical for septic shock (e.g. approximately three quarters had normal blood lactate levels). (2) We have no information about protocol compliance with PALS resuscitation guidelines in the control group. For example, the median fluid resuscitation in the first 6-hour postrandomisation was only 5 mL/kg, suggesting noncompliance. (3) The incidence of the primary target for EGDT, venous hypoxia, was low in both groups, and did not differ at baseline or 6 hours, with no difference in absolute values of venous saturation at any time point. (4) There were no differences in days of mechanical ventilation, inotrope use or PICU stay. (5) The timing of mortality for the majority of the control group occurred after day 14, well beyond PICU discharge, and atypical for that seen in most PICUs.

A further limitation of EGDT for children is the requirement for superior vena caval access, which is highly likely to necessitate intubation and ventilation. This is because femoral venous lines are more susceptible to regional tissue bed variation in venous saturation, dependent upon where the line tip sits (e.g. renal vein saturations are typically in the 90s, producing a potential false negative result).

Fluid resuscitation

The surviving sepsis guidelines for children recommend repeated 20 mL/kg boluses of isotonic crystalloids or albumin equivalent with reassessment, up to 60 mL/kg; at which point catecholamines should be commenced [2]. This practice has recently been called into question from a minority of UK clinicians, following the 'fluid expansion as supportive therapy' (FEAST) trial [8] in 2011. This large (n = 3141), pragmatic, African RCT evaluated whether repeated boluses (up to 40 mL/kg) of either normal saline or 5% albumin at presentation to hospital improved mortality in children with severe infection, compared to standard care (no bolus). The trial was stopped after an interim analysis showed an excess mortality at 48 hours in both treatment arms compared to controls (10.5% versus 7.3%). This trial was of a very high quality, but illustrates the danger of extrapolating findings beyond the settings outlined by the patients, intervention, comparator, outcome format (PICO).

The FEAST patient population is very dissimilar to developed world populations. Children in developing countries generally present later with illness (early recognition and treatment being perhaps the most important element of the sepsis bundle). Patients in the FEAST trial exhibited a high rate of severe anaemia (one third had a haemoglobin <5 g/dL), 57% had malaria, and only 39/3170 had severe hypotension [8]. The intervention was not comparable: fluid boluses limited to 40 mL/kg total is not seen as sufficient in the developed world if hypoperfusion persists. The comparator group did not receive ongoing monitoring at a frequency considered mandatory in developed countries (pulse oximetry, heart rate and blood pressure checks were documented at 1, 4, 8, 24 and 48 hours), and more advanced therapies (such as intensive care) are unavailable.

The mechanism of harm in the FEAST trial is, as yet, undetermined. The authors undertook a rigorous set of subgroup analyses (including malaria and severe anaemia), and did not show any heterogeneity of effect. They suggested that 'the vasoconstrictor response in shock confers protection by reducing perfusion to nonvital tissues, and rapid reversal with fluid resuscitation is deleterious' [8]. Thus, rather than FEAST calling into question current fluid resuscitation practice in the developed world, it has highlighted the problems of partial resuscitation in a resource poor setting.

Early empiric antibiotic therapy

Appropriate (right drug, right dose and right time) antibiotic administration appears to confer a consistent survival benefit in paediatric and adult observational studies [9,10].

Adherence to bundles

A care process will only be adopted if it is clinically acceptable and can be performed in the majority of clinical settings. Although the sepsis bundle meets these requirements, it has been shown that uptake requires sustained effort: in bundle-naïve adult settings, adherence may only rise from 10% at baseline to 55% a year later, despite a concerted teaching programme [11]. Paediatric evidence also points towards poor compliance with guidelines. A part of the problem may be lack of awareness, e.g. the American College of Critical Care PALS guidelines were initially published only in a critical care journal, despite the fact that the majority of first-line resuscitating clinicians are paediatricians, emergency medicine practitioners and anaesthetists. A French PICU survey found generally high perceived compliance, apart from targeting central venous pressure and utilising insulin to achieve tight glucose control (discussed later in the chapter) [12]. There is clearly more work to do in this area.

Catheter associated blood stream infections and quality improvement

Catheter associated blood stream infections (CA-BSI) carry significant morbidity and mortality on PICU. In 2003, the keystone intensive care unit project [13] was launched in Michigan, USA, as a safety initiative to reduce CA-BSI. The project targeted five key areas of practice associated with the insertion and management of central venous catheters: hand-washing technique, use of barrier precautions, chlorhexidine skin decontamination, avoidance of femoral vein and early catheter removal. In the 103 intensive care units that took part, the mean rate of CA-BSI decreased from 7.7 to 1.4 per 1000 catheter days, which was sustained at 3-year follow-up [14].

Based on these compelling results, the UK National Patient Safety Agency announced a national initiative known as 'Matching Michigan' [15]. The programme ran for 2 years between 2009 and 2011, receiving data returns from 215/223 intensive care units in England (196 adult, 19 paediatric). Of note, paediatric CA-BSIs accounted for 14.6% of total declared infections, but only 7.89% of total catheter days. Overall, CA-BSI halved, although this did not reach statistical significance in paediatric patients (5.7–2.9 per 1000 catheter days, P = 0.6), compared to adults (3.7–1.5, P < 0.0001); this was likely due to being underpowered.

Matching Michigan highlighted the burden of CA-BSI in PICU and emphasised the potential for health care improvement with systemwide changes in practice [15]. However, caution is needed in ascribing causation entirely to the 'Matching Michigan' initiative, as this took place against a backdrop of political and media pressure to reduce hospital-acquired infections, whereby a range of other measures were introduced into health care systems (alcohol gel availability for visitors to the ward, antimicrobial stewardship, infection rates as financial incentives, etc.).

Possible explanations for the discrepancy between adult and paediatric infection rates have been suggested, including smaller veins which are more predisposed to thrombosis and bacterial adhesion, greater use of the femoral venous route and a lower frequency of line replacement [16]. The Catheter Infections in Children Study [17] was designed to address some of these issues. This UK-based RCT took place in 14 PICUs, enrolling over 1400 patients, who were randomised to receive one of three catheter types: standard, heparin-bonded or antibiotic impregnated. Study recruitment is complete and, at time of writing, results are imminent.

THERAPEUTIC HYPOTHERMIA

The use of therapeutic hypothermia (TH) as a brain-protective strategy post-cardiac arrest was first suggested in the 1950s, following increasing intraoperative utilisation with cardiac surgery. However, between 1960 and 1990, the use of TH decreased due to perceived complications and the resources available to manage these. The 1990s witnessed a resurgence of interest in TH, following animal studies that showed better outcomes postcerebral hypoxic insult, and the development of new techniques for studying the brain [18]. To date, most studies utilise a target temperature of 33°C (32–34°C), with differences in the time windows for induction and maintenance.

Neonatal use of TH for early treatment of hypoxic ischaemic encephalopathy was evaluated over the last decade with publication of several key trials. A landmark RCT, published in 2009, was the Total Body Hypothermia for Neonatal Encephalopathy (TOBY) trial [19]. Although there was no difference in the primary outcome (combined risk of death or severe disability at 18 months), the TOBY trial revealed TH benefit in terms of survival without neurologic abnormality. This benefit is sustained through to early childhood and as such [20], TH is now standard of care for neonates with hypoxic ischaemic encephalopathy.

In adult medicine, two landmark papers were published in 2002 [21,22], demonstrating benefit of TH in terms of both hospital survival and neurological outcome after cardiac arrest with ventricular fibrillation. Although both studies were relatively small, the International Liaison Committee on Resuscitation (ILCOR) felt the evidence strong enough to update the 2003 guidelines, recommending TH in adults postventricular fibrillation cardiac arrest [23]. Following this, on the basis of growing neonatal and adult evidence and a relatively favourable safety profile, the 2006 guidelines recommended TH consideration in comatose children after cardiac arrest [24].

Utilisation of TH following paediatric cardiac arrest remains sporadic, with a 2010 survey of UK paediatric intensivists reporting that <50% of respondents 'always or often' using it, with 'lack of evidence' cited as the commonest reason [25]. This is further underlined by the mechanism of cardiac arrest being different in paediatrics where asystole and pulseless electrical activity are more common than ventricular fibrillation or ventricular tachycardia.

There is growing evidence that fever in the postarrest period is detrimental [26]. This has led some to speculate that the apparent benefits of TH may not be due to cooling per se, but rather due to the avoidance of hyperthermia. This is consistent with re-examination of the landmark TH trials (both adult and neonatal), where fever was common in the control groups. In the adult study [22], approximately one quarter of hourly temperature measurements in the control group were >38.0°C for the 36-hour postenrolment. In the TOBY trial [19], 14% of control neonates manifested a rectal temperature >38.0°C on at least two occasions.

To address this, Nielson et al [27] conducted a targeted temperature management trial, the largest (n = 950) adult multicentre RCT to date. Patients were randomised to 'active temperature control' for 24 hours at 33°C versus normothermia at 36°C. Here, the probability of a control patient exhibiting a temperature >38.0°C within the first 24 hours was <10%, and this was almost never sustained beyond 1-hour duration. The results showed similar mortality rates in both groups (50% versus 48%).

From this, some concluded that cooling patients to 36°C is equivalent to 33°C and suggested aiming for this 'normothermic' target. However, the trial was not an equivalence study but was designed to detect a 20% difference between groups (with 80% power) and, therefore, failed to prove a difference in therapies. At present, ILCOR have not changed their guidelines and continue to support hypothermia at 32–34°C. As debate continues, it is interesting to note that the rates of complications between groups in the targeted temperature management trial were the same, and that maintaining 'normothermia' still required active temperature management systems.

Paediatric-specific evidence

The TH after paediatric cardiac arrest (THAPCA) trials [28] was commenced in 2009, comparing TH (32–34°C) with normothermia (36–37.5°C) for 48 hours after cardiac arrest. Two THAPCA trials are being performed: one (completed, but not reported) examines out-of-hospital cardiac arrest, the second (due for completion in 2015) in-hospital arrest. These studies were in planning for over 10 years and are a stark reminder of the complexities of conducting research in PICU. It is hoped that these will provide a definitive answer for TH in PICU.

TIGHT GLYCAEMIC CONTROL

Arguably, the therapy with the greatest impact in the last 15 years to have 'come and gone' across the intensive care environment is insulin for tight glycaemic control (TGC). Hyperglycaemia associated with insulin resistance has long been recognised in critically ill patients and thought to represent an adaptive, stress response [29]. This notion was challenged in 2001 with the hypothesis that hyperglycaemia may increase mortality and complications in critical illness. Van den Berghe et al published a single centre trial of TGC in a surgical intensive care unit in Leuven, utilising insulin to maintain blood glucose at 4.4–6.1 mmol/L (intensive group) versus 10.0–11.1 mmol/L (control) [29]. The trial was stopped early (n = 1548) after an interim analysis showed that the risk of intensive care unit mortality was 8% in the control group versus 4.6% in the TGC group ($P < 0.04$). There were also dramatic differences favouring TGC in the secondary outcomes, including rate of blood stream infections and need for blood transfusion.

These were remarkable results from a relatively cheap and widely available therapy. Many hospitals swiftly adopted TGC and even promoted TGC compliance as a marker of quality of care. However, criticisms were raised about safety (potential for hypoglycaemia) and the validity and generalisability of these results. In particular, the feeding regime in Leuven resulted in a very high utilisation of total parenteral nutrition (more than was used at that time elsewhere). As a consequence, the 2004 Surviving Sepsis Guidelines recommended a less rigid version of TGC (aiming for blood glucose <8.3 mmol/L), and recommended commencing enteral feeding as soon as possible.

A follow-up trial [30] from Leuven in medical patients failed to show a mortality benefit (40% versus 37.3%); however, TGC again appeared to be beneficial across similar secondary endpoints. Here, the incidence of hypoglycaemia was much higher with TGC (19% versus 3%).

Over the following decade, a number of multicentre studies were published: none replicated the Leuven results, and several suggested harm. In 2008, a factorial trial was published by Brunkhorst et al [31], whereby TGC was evaluated concurrently with the choice of fluid resuscitation in sepsis. The TGC limb was terminated early (n = 488) because of concern over hypoglycaemia (17% versus 4.1%). The Normoglycemia in Intensive Care Evaluation-Survival Using Glucose Algorithm Regulation (NICE-SUGAR) [32] study is the largest TGC study to date, randomising 6104 patients in 42 intensive care units (Australia, New Zealand and Canada). There was no difference in the primary outcome (90-day mortality), which was 27.5% in the intensive group versus 24.9% in standard care. Again there were more severe episodes of hypoglycaemia in the intervention group (6.8% versus 0.5%).

One large neonatal study [33] (n = 389) has evaluated TGC in very low-birth-weight infants. Similar to the adult RCTs, there were no differences in the primary (mortality) or secondary outcomes, and a higher incidence of hypoglycaemia in the TGC arm (29% versus 17%).

Paediatric-specific evidence

The Leuven group also published in 2009 the first TGC trial in children, enrolling 700 patients [34]. Although not the primary outcome, TGC again showed a mortality benefit, similar to the original adult trial by this group (6% versus 3%). Similar to the adult experience, two subsequent large multicentre RCTs did not show benefit. The first, a 2-centre, US study following cardiac surgery (n = 980) exhibited similar health care associated infections (8.6 versus 9.9 per 1000 patient days, $P = 0.67$) [35]. The second, was a 13-centre (n = 1369) UK-based study by Macrae et al [Control of Hyperglycaemia in Paediatric intensive care (CHIP) trial] [36]. Here, TGC targeted a blood glucose of 4.0–7.0 mmol/L, with the control target being <12 mmol/L. The mean between-group difference in the number of days alive and free from mechanical ventilation at 30 days was 0.36 days [95% confidence interval (CI), -0.42 to 1.14]. Severe hypoglycaemia occurred in a higher proportion of children in the TGC group (7.3% versus 1.5%), in keeping with the largest adult study [32].

The story of TGC is a cautionary tale of evidence-based medicine in our time. It reminds us that all single centre studies require external, multicentre validation, particularly when stopped early for benefit. However, on the plus side, it is an example of the progress made in PICU research, which has allowed us to draw firm conclusions for paediatric patients: TGC in PICU does not improve mortality or clinically important secondary outcomes and increases the risk of harm to patients.

HIGH-FREQUENCY OSCILLATION VENTILATION

The potential for positive pressure ventilation to damage the lung (ventilator-induced lung injury) is well documented. The mechanism is thought to be a combination of lung over distension, excessive pressure and shearing forces caused by cyclical closing and opening of alveoli. Over the past 20 years, high-frequency oscillation ventilation (HFOV) was thought to offer better lung protection compared to conventional, intermittent positive pressure ventilation; and has become the default therapy in many PICUs for diffuse, severe lung disease. However, this is based largely upon theoretical physiological principles, without a strong evidence base for efficacy.

Neonatal practitioners pioneered HFOV use, primarily in respiratory distress syndrome. A 2009 Cochrane review [37] comparing HFOV with conventional ventilation evaluated 17 trials (n = 3652), of which 9 trials (n = 2060) had the primary endpoint of 28-day mortality, and 6 (n = 1043) evaluated the presence of chronic lung disease at 28–30 days in survivors; no between group difference was found for either endpoint. To date, there has been only one RCT of HFOV in paediatric practice, published 20 years ago. Arnold et al [38] randomised 70 patients with 'diffuse alveolar disease' to conventional ventilation versus HFOV at five PICUs. There was no difference in mortality between groups but they did report a significantly lower need for supplemental oxygen at 30 days in the HFOV group.

Adult practice was slower to adopt HFOV; however, initial data suggested some benefit over conventional ventilation in ARDS. A 2013 Cochrane review evaluated six RCTs published in 2002–2007, and showed a 23% relative reduction in 30-day mortality with HFOV [39]. However, the review authors acknowledged many of these studies used suboptimal practice in terms of conventional ventilation. For example, three utilised tidal volumes in excess of the recommended 6–8 mL/kg, which can exacerbate lung damage and increase mortality [40]. Interestingly, subgroup analysis of the neonatal trials also suggested HFOV benefit when lung protective conventional ventilation was not used [37].

Shortly after the Cochrane review, two large, well-designed multicentre RCTs were published which utilised a lung-protective strategy in the conventional ventilation arms, by limiting tidal volumes and plateau pressures, and optimising positive end expiratory pressure. The high frequency Oscillation in Ards (OSCAR) trial (n = 795) found very similar mortality in the conventional and HFOV groups (41.1% versus 41.7%) [41]. The oscillation for acute respiratory distress syndrome treated early (OSCILLATE) study was stopped early because of increased mortality (47% versus 35%) in the HFOV group [42]. The reason for the differing mortality between groups is unclear. In both studies, patients in the HFOV groups received increased amounts of sedatives and muscle relaxants. The OSCAR study allowed for a wider variation in HFOV protocol and had a lower mean airway pressure [41], with less haemodynamic compromise which perhaps offered some protection.

These trials have not negated HFOV as a valid therapy for lung support [41,42], but perhaps refocussed us on the need to use both conventional ventilation and HFOV wisely, as both can cause lung damage. Definitive paediatric HFOV trials are still awaited.

CONCLUSION

A recurring theme of this review has been the introduction of a range of therapies which initially showed promise, but were subsequently shown to be nonbeneficial. However, rather than viewing these negative findings with disappointment, they have illustrated several important concepts, as discussed below:

1   It is important to get the basics right. A novel therapy may seem beneficial largely because 'standard care' is actually nonstandardised. However, the latter has less to do with research design, and is more about efficient organisation of health care systems.

2. Trial design and delivery is improving; the multicentre RCT has come of age in PICU, particularly, in the United Kingdom. However, improved PICU outcomes pose a challenge for evaluating new therapies. Thus, we need to continue to refine trial design by asking clear, simple questions, exploring new endpoints and considering alternative designs (e.g. factorial trials).

3. There is great potential for shared learning with our adult and neonatal colleagues. A remarkable finding has been similarity of results across the intensive care spectrum with the evaluation of many key therapies.

It is hoped that these principles will be applied to the development and evaluation of current and future therapies in the intensive care environment.

Key points for clinical practice

- Improvements in paediatric intensive care within the last two decades have been driven largely by better health care organisation and standardisation of existing therapies, and not introduction of novel therapies.

- Clinical trial design and conduct are better. In addition, many similar therapies are now evaluated across neonatal, paediatric and adult intensive care environments, creating potential for maximising knowledge transfer.

- The improvement in 'standard care' and better clinical trial evaluation has largely negated the apparent benefit of many advanced therapies.

REFERENCES

1. Paediatric Intensive Care Audit Network. PICANET. Available from: http://www.picanet.org.uk. [Last accessed 18 November 2014.]
2. Dellinger RP, Levy MM, Rhodes A, et al. Surviving sepsis campaign: international guidelines for management of severe sepsis and septic shock: 2012. Crit Care Med 2013; 4:580–637.
3. Rivers E, Nguyen B, Havstad S, et al. Early goal-directed therapy in the treatment of severe sepsis and septic shock. N Engl J Med 2001; 345:1368–1377.
4. The ARISE Investigators and the ANZICS Clinical Trials Group. Goal-directed resuscitation for patients with early septic shock. N Engl J Med 2014; 371:1496–1506.
5. The ProCESS Investigators, Yealy DM, Kellum JA, et al. A randomized trial of protocol-based care for early septic shock. N Engl J Med 2014; 370:1683–1693.
6. Han YY, Carcillo JA, Dragotta MA, et al. Early reversal of pediatric-neonatal septic shock by community physicians is associated with improved outcome. Pediatrics 2003; 112:793–799.
7. De Oliveira CF, de Oliveira DSF, Gottschald AFC, et al. ACCM/PALS haemodynamic support guidelines for paediatric septic shock: an outcomes comparison with and without monitoring central venous oxygen saturation. Intensive Care Med 2008; 34:1065–1075.
8. Maitland K, Kiguli S, Opoka RO, et al. Mortality after fluid bolus in African children with severe infection. N Engl J Med 2011; 364:2483–2495.
9. Ferrer R, Martin-Loeches I, Phillips G, et al. Empiric antibiotic treatment reduces mortality in severe sepsis and septic shock from the first hour: results from a guideline-based performance improvement program. Crit Care Med 2014; 42:1749–1755.
10. Weiss SL, Fitzgerald JC, Balamuth F, et al. Delayed antimicrobial therapy increases mortality and organ dysfunction duration in pediatric sepsis. Crit Care Med 2014; 42:2409–2417.
11. Nguyen HB, Kuan WS, Batech M, et al. Outcome effectiveness of the severe sepsis resuscitation bundle with addition of lactate clearance as a bundle item: a multi-national evaluation. Crit Care 2011; 15:R229.
12. Santschi M, Leclerc F. Management of children with sepsis and septic shock: a survey among pediatric intensivists of the Réseau Mère-Enfant de la Francophonie. Ann Intensive Care 2013; 3:7.
13. Pronovost P, Needham D, Berenholtz S, et al. An intervention to decrease catheter-related bloodstream infections in the ICU. N Engl J Med 2006; 355:2725–2732.
14. Pronovost PJ, Goeschel CA, Colantuoni E, et al. Sustaining reductions in catheter related bloodstream infections in Michigan intensive care units: observational study. BMJ 2010; 340:c309.
15. Bion J, Richardson A, Hibbert P, et al. 'Matching Michigan': a 2-year stepped interventional programme to minimise central venous catheter-blood stream infections in intensive care units in England. BMJ Qual Saf 2013; 22:110–123.
16. Mok Q, Gilbert R. Interventions to reduce central venous catheter-associated infections in children: which ones are beneficial? Intensive Care Med 2011; 37:566–568.
17. CATCH Trial Team. Catheter infections in children. Available from: http://www.catchtrial.org.uk. [Last accessed 18 November 2014.]
18. Varon J. Therapeutic hypothermia: past, present, and future. Chest 2008; 133:1267–1274.
19. Azzopardi DV, Strohm B, Edwards AD, et al. Moderate hypothermia to treat perinatal asphyxial encephalopathy. N Engl J Med 2009; 361:1349–1358.
20. Azzopardi D, Strohm B, Marlow N, et al. Effects of hypothermia for perinatal asphyxia on childhood outcomes. N Engl J Med 2014; 371:140–149.
21. Bernard SA, Gray TW, Buist MD, et al. Treatment of comatose survivors of out-of-hospital cardiac arrest with induced hypothermia. N Engl J Med 2002; 346:557–563.
22. Hypothermia after Cardiac Arrest Study Group. Mild therapeutic hypothermia to improve the neurologic outcome after cardiac arrest. N Engl J Med 2002; 346:549–556.
23. Nolan JP. Therapeutic hypothermia after cardiac arrest: an advisory statement by the advanced life support task force of the International Liaison Committee on Resuscitation. Circulation 2003; 108:118–121.
24. The International Liaison Committee on Resuscitation. The International Liaison Committee on Resuscitation (ILCOR) consensus on science with treatment recommendations for pediatric and neonatal patients: pediatric basic and advanced life support. Pediatrics 2006; 117:e955–e977.
25. Scholefield BR, Duncan HP, Morris KP. Survey of the use of therapeutic hypothermia post cardiac arrest. Arch Dis Child 2010; 95:796–799.
26. Leary M, Grossestreuer AV, Iannacone S, et al. Pyrexia and neurologic outcomes after therapeutic hypothermia for cardiac arrest. Resuscitation 2013; 84:1056–1061.

27. Nielsen N, Wetterslev J, Cronberg T, et al. Targeted temperature management at 33°C versus 36°C after cardiac arrest. N Engl J Med 2013; 369:2197–2206.
28. Moler FW, Silverstein FS, Meert KL, et al. Rationale, timeline, study design, and protocol overview of the therapeutic hypothermia after pediatric cardiac arrest trials. Pediatr Crit Care Med 2013; 14:e304–e315.
29. Van Den Berghe G, Wouters P, Weekers F, et al. Intensive insulin therapy in critically ill patients. N Engl J Med 2001; 345:1359–1367.
30. Van den Berghe G, Wilmer A, Hermans G, et al. Intensive insulin therapy in the medical ICU. N Engl J Med 2006; 354:449.
31. Brunkhorst FM, Engel C, Bloos F, et al. Intensive insulin therapy and pentastarch resuscitation in severe sepsis. N Engl J Med 2008; 358:125–139.
32. Finfer S, Chittock DR, Su SY-S, et al. Intensive versus conventional glucose control in critically ill patients. N Engl J Med 2009; 360:1283–1297.
33. Beardsall K, Vanhaesebrouck S, Ogilvy-Stuart AL, et al. Early insulin therapy in very-low-birth-weight infants. N Engl J Med 2008; 359:1873–1884.
34. Vlasselaers D, Milants I, Desmet L, et al. Intensive insulin therapy for patients in paediatric intensive care: a prospective, randomised controlled study. Lancet 2009; 373:547–556.
35. Agus MSD, Steil GM, Wypij D, et al. Tight glycemic control versus standard care after pediatric cardiac surgery. N Engl J Med 2012; 367:1208–1219.
36. Macrae D, Grieve R, Allen E, et al. A randomized trial of hyperglycemic control in pediatric intensive care. N Engl J Med 2014; 370:107–118.
37. Cools F, Henderson-Smart DJ, Offringa M, et al. Elective high frequency oscillatory ventilation versus conventional ventilation for acute pulmonary dysfunction in preterm infants. Cochrane Database Syst Rev 2009; 3:CD000104.
38. Arnold JH, Hanson JH, Toro-Figuero LO, et al. Prospective, randomized comparison of high-frequency oscillatory ventilation and conventional mechanical ventilation in pediatric respiratory failure. Crit Care Med 1994; 22:1530–1539.
39. Sud S, Sud M, Friedrich JO, et al. High-frequency ventilation versus conventional ventilation for treatment of acute lung injury and acute respiratory distress syndrome. Cochrane Database Syst Rev 2013; 2:CD004085.
40. The Acute Respiratory Distress Syndrome Network. Ventilation with lower tidal volumes as compared with traditional tidal volumes for acute lung injury and the acute respiratory distress syndrome. N Engl J Med 2000; 342:1302–1308.
41. Young D, Lamb SE, Shah S, et al. High-frequency oscillation for acute respiratory distress syndrome. N Engl J Med 2013; 368:806–813.
42. Ferguson ND, Cook DJ, Guyatt GH, et al. High-frequency oscillation in early acute respiratory distress syndrome. N Engl J Med 2013; 368:795–805.

Chapter 9

Intranasal medicines in paediatrics

Danielle S Hall, Ian Chi Kei Wong,

INTRODUCTION

Intranasal drug administration has been used in clinical paediatric practice since the 1980s [1], but the intranasal route dates back thousands of years to India [2]. Currently, it is most commonly used in paediatrics to provide opiate relief in painful sickle cell crises, long bone fractures, burns, and is used in almost two thirds of paediatric emergency departments in England and Wales [3]. There are many other applications for intranasal medications, including sedation, rescue therapy in prolonged seizures, migraine relief and vaccine administration. This chapter will discuss the advantages and disadvantages of the intranasal route of drug administration, current evidence for common intranasal medications used in children and its future applications in paediatrics.

WHY INTRANASAL?

Nasal anatomy, pharmacodynamics and delivery devices

Painful administration of medication to children risks poor adherence and a negative attitude towards health professionals. Children do not like needles and describe venepuncture as one of their most frightening hospital experiences [4]. In general, oral medications have a slow onset of action because they are metabolised via the hepatic first-pass pathway. Unlike the oral route, intranasally administered medicines bypass first-pass metabolism, increasing their bioavailability [2]. This confers a major advantage when a rapid effect is required, such as cases with severe pain or seizure activity.

Entry to the nasal cavity is via the nasal vestibule, otherwise known as the nostrils. The internal surface area of the nasal cavity is increased by the turbinates, three extensions of tissue from the nasal wall. The nasal mucosa offers a surface area with a highly vascularised blood supply; blood flow per cubic centimetre is higher than even muscle, brain or liver [5]. The pH of the nasal mucosa in a child is between 5.0 and 6.7 [6]. Thus, lipophilic drugs with a neutral pH and small molecular weight of up to 1000 Da^2 dissolve in the nasal mucosal

Danielle S Hall MA Oxon MBBS MRCPCH FHEA, Paediatric Emergency Medicine, St Thomas' Hospital, London, UK. Email: dani.hall@doctors.org.uk (for correspondence)

Ian Chi Kei Wong PhD FRCPCH FRPharmS, Centre for Paediatric Pharmacy Research, Research Department of Practice and Policy, UCL School of Pharmacy, London, UK layer, passing through the epithelium into the blood stream by passive transcellular and paracellular diffusion [6].

Venous drainage from the nose passes into the internal jugular vein, draining to the right side of the heart via the superior vena cava. The blood is then pumped to the lungs, passing back into the left side of the heart to be pumped into the systemic circulation. There is a theoretical possibility, the nose to brain theory, that some centrally acting drugs with a very small particle size of <10 μm can drift to the very back of the nasal cavity to the olfactory bulb and pass directly into the central nervous system via the olfactory nerve [7]. The nasal cavity and surrounding tissues are illustrated in **Figure 9.1**.

It is important that only small volumes of drug are used. Large volumes result in a phenomenon known as 'dripping'. The drug may drip anteriorly out of the nose or run off posteriorly to the oropharynx and then be swallowed, thus absorbed via the gut and subjected to first-pass metabolism. Then effects of the drug can be less predictable. The optimal characteristics of an intranasal drug are summarised in **Table 9.1**.

There are three methods described for intranasal drug administration. Simply dripping the drug from a syringe into the nostril is the most commonly method used in paediatric emergency departments in England and Wales [3]. Apparatus is also available in the form of a spray device attached to the end of a syringe, or specially manufactured mucosal atomising devices which reduce particle droplet size and increase the mucosal area over which the drug is delivered, increasing bioavailability [4]. Evidence suggests that drugs delivered via an atomising device have a greater efficacy than when dripped from a syringe as this reduces run-off of the drug to the oropharynx [1].

The advantages and disadvantages of the intranasal route of administration in paediatric practice are summarised in **Table 9.2**.

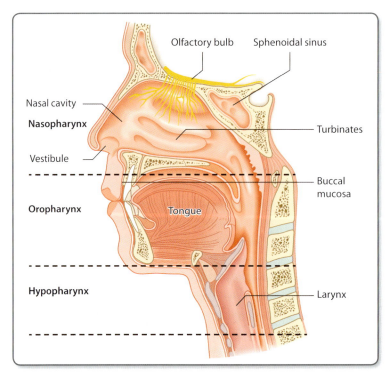

Figure 9.1 Cross section of the nose and surrounding structures.

Olfactory bulb   Sphenoidal sinus

Nasal cavity

Nasopharynx

Vestibule

Turbinates

Buccal mucosa

Oropharynx   Tongue

Hypopharynx   Larynx

Table 9.1 Optimal characteristics for intranasal drugs
Small molecular weights of up to 1000 Da
Highly lipophilic to optimise absorption across cell membranes
Water soluble to aid pharmaceutical formulation
Small volume between 50 and 250 µL [34]
Neutral pH

Table 9.2 Advantages and disadvantages of the intranasal route of drug administration

Advantages	Disadvantages
High patient and provider satisfaction	Limited to drugs with a maximal volume of between 50 and 250 µL
Highly acceptable to children	Nasal irritation
No-needle technique reducing iatrogenic pain	May be contraindicated in certain conditions
Can be administered by parents or carers at home	Nasal absorption may be retarded in conditions with impedance of nasociliary action such as cystic fibrosis and Karteneger's syndrome [6]
Children over 9 years of age can self-administer [35]	Reduction of nasal mucosal surface, e.g. in epistaxis, reduces the area for drug absorption [1]
Rapid onset of action as first-pass metabolism is bypassed	
Increased bioavailability compared to orally administered drugs	
Possible direct access to the central nervous system	
Despite concerns that coryza, a very common symptom in children, would impede absorption due to increased mucous production, this does not appear to be the case [36]	

CURRENT APPLICATIONS IN PAEDIATRICS

The intranasal route of administration is used commonly in paediatrics. A recent survey of paediatric emergency departments in England and Wales revealed that most departments are using intranasal diamorphine and/or midazolam [3]. The most common applications of intranasal drugs in paediatrics are for analgesia, rescue anticonvulsant therapy and sedation, although other applications are also available. The following section will examine the evidence for each of these categories of drugs.

Opiate analgesia

Children with severe pain, e.g. due to fractures or painful sickle cell crises, need effective, fast-acting analgesia. An ideal analgesic provides effective pain relief with a rapid onset of action and is painless to administer. Absorption rates and bioavailability of oral analgesia can be unpredictable [8]. Despite intravenous opiates being effective at managing pain in children, placing intravenous lines is both painful and may delay drug administration. Intranasal opiate administration is less traumatic than giving opiates via the intravenous route and the onset of action may be quicker in comparison to intravenous morphine [4]. This has been addressed by the Royal College of Emergency Medicine who have produced clinical standards for the management of children in moderate or severe pain arriving at emergency departments [9]. This guideline recommends that children in severe pain are treated with either intranasal diamorphine 0.1 mg/kg made up to 0.2 mL, intravenous morphine or both. Many countries outside the United Kingdom have limited access to diamorphine, using intranasal fentanyl instead. There have been no direct comparisons of intranasal diamorphine and fentanyl, so it is not clear if one is superior to the other.

Sixty per cent of emergency departments in England and Wales use intranasal diamorphine to treat pain in children [10]. It is highly acceptable to children and parents [11]. Diamorphine is a derivative of morphine, made by acetylation, and when given intranasally to children it exhibits an excellent safety profile [10]. It is an extremely water-soluble drug, so can easily be formulated into a preparation suitable for intranasal administration, with peak plasma concentrations reached within approximately 5 minutes [3]. Compared to intramuscular morphine, pain scores improve significantly faster after intranasal diamorphine [3]. In a retrospective case series comparing intranasal diamorphine with intravenous morphine, children who received intranasal diamorphine were less likely to require further analgesia while in the emergency department [10]. Intranasal diamorphine can also be safely combined with oral morphine, obviating the need for further intravenous opiates [11].

Fentanyl is a highly selective synthetic opioid agonist that does not cause histamine release, resulting in fewer cardiorespiratory effects than other opiates. When given intranasally, the onset is within 2–3 minutes, with effects lasting up to half an hour [4]. When given via a mucosal atomising device in doses of 1.5 µg/kg, children with severe pain experience a substantial reduction in pain score at 5 and 30 minutes postadministration [8]. A systematic review published in 2011 of the available literature on intranasal fentanyl showed that intranasal fentanyl results in significant improvement in pain score in children within 10 minutes of administration and is an effective alternative to morphine in alleviating painful fractures and burns in children [4]. It is, therefore, unsurprising that parents prefer intranasal fentanyl to intramuscular morphine [4].

There is emerging evidence that intranasal naloxone might be an effective alternative to intravenous naloxone in adults to reverse the effects of the respiratory and central nervous system caused by opiates [7]. This is supported by reports that paramedics in the United States administer naloxone intranasally to reduce their risk of needle stick injury when treating patients suffering from opiate overdose, a population at high risk for blood-borne viruses in whom vascular access may be challenging [7]. Intranasal naloxone may also be a viable medication for use in paediatrics.

Triptans in acute migraine

Another application of intranasal analgesia in children is for the treatment of acute migraine. Migraine is a common complaint in childhood with a significant impact on school attendance. The mainstay treatment for paediatric acute migraine is simple nonsteroidal analgesia or 5-hydroxytriptamine receptor agonists, also known as triptans. The most commonly used triptan is sumatriptan. Oral triptans exhibit variable and sometimes unpredictable clinical effects which may be secondary to gastrointestinal phenomena experienced in migraine such as delayed gastric emptying [12]. There is no evidence for or against the use of oral or subcutaneous sumatriptan. A systematic literature review of the evidence for intranasal sumatriptan in children, published in 2013, showed that intranasal sumatriptan is an effective treatment for migraine in adolescents [12]. Most of the published research on intranasal sumatriptan compares its use to placebo, which is complicated by the fact that large placebo effects are seen in children and adolescents with migraine. Nonetheless, the systematic review showed that intranasal sumatriptan produces better headache relief and complete headache resolution 2 hours after treatment and is more efficacious in comparison to placebo [12]. Intranasal sumatriptan is also effective at relieving the nonheadache symptoms of vomiting and photophobia that can be associated with migraine. Commonly quoted doses of intranasal sumatriptan are 10 mg in children <40 kg in weight and 20 mg for children >40 kg. However, there has been no direct comparison of intranasal triptans and simple nonsteroidal treatment, so whether one is superior to the other in treating children migraines currently remains unclear.

Benzodiazepine anticonvulsants

Seizures are common in children. The primary goal of anticonvulsant rescue therapy is to terminate a seizure to prevent hypoxia and secondary neurological and systemic compromise. Historically, rectal diazepam has been used as the first-line treatment for children in whom no venous access is available. Now, however, there is considerable evidence that intranasal benzodiazepines may be a superior alternative as well as being a more socially acceptable route of administration by carers and teachers in the community [13].

Midazolam is highly lipophilic at physiological pH with a low molecular weight of 325.8 Da and is therefore easily absorbed through the nasal mucosa and blood brain barrier. It attenuates γ-aminobutyric acid activity, a major inhibitory neurotransmitter. When given intranasally, it reaches maximal plasma concentration within 12 minutes with a volume of distribution double that of intravenous midazolam [13].

Although the rectum is highly vascularised allowing rapid absorption of drugs into the blood stream, rectal medications do not bypass hepatic first-pass metabolism; hence the onset of action is delayed compared to drugs given intranasally [14]. Rectal absorption may be highly variable with wide ranging bioavailability [13]. Furthermore, cumulative doses of rectal benzodiazepines are associated with a high risk of respiratory depression [14].

A literature review published in 2013 illustrated that, when directly compared to rectal diazepam, intranasal midazolam given in doses of 0.2 mg/kg divided between the two nostrils terminates seizures significantly more quickly (1.95 minutes versus 2.97 minutes) and more reliably than rectal diazepam with a lesser need for hospitalisation or paediatric intensive care unit admission [13]. Intranasal midazolam also has a better side-effect profile than rectal diazepam; it is less likely to cause a drop in oxygen saturations, vomiting or excessive drowsiness [13].

An alternative to intranasal midazolam is buccal midazolam. Drugs administered via the buccal mucosa are absorbed via the lining of the cheeks, gums and lips, bypassing first-pass hepatic metabolism in the same way as intranasal drugs do. NICE, the National Institute for Clinical Excellence, issued a guideline in 2012 recommending buccal midazolam as a first-line treatment for status epilepticus in the prehospital setting [15]. Like intranasal midazolam, buccal midazolam has a quicker onset of action than rectal diazepam with a similar safety profile [16].

Status epilepticus algorithms recommend giving intravenous lorazepam to a fitting child if venous access is available. However, there has also been evidence published which may suggest that intranasal lorazepam is an acceptable alternative to intravenous lorazepam, with a similar efficacy in terms of seizure cessation with a good safety profile [17].

Sedation

Benzodiazepines are commonly used to sedate children for painful or frightening procedures. An ideal sedative for children would have a rapid onset and recovery time, titratable effects to dose, be painless to administer with no significant adverse events. Midazolam is the most commonly used benzodiazepine for procedural sedation in children, acting as an anxiolytic and amnesic. It is given intranasally in doses of 0.2–0.4 mg/kg and has been shown to be efficacious at producing sedation; compared to oral and buccal administration, aerosolised intranasal midazolam has the most rapid onset of action and highest rate of successful sedation, and is most favoured by parents for laceration repair [18]. It is also used successfully as a preanaesthetic for children undergoing general anaesthesia [18]. However, as midazolam is only water soluble at a low pH of 3–3.5, it stimulates pain receptors in the trigeminal nerve when given intranasally [3] and is not tolerated well by children [18].

Recently, intranasal dexmedetomidine has made an appearance in the literature as an effective sedative in children. It is a selective $\alpha2$ adrenoreceptor agonist resulting in sedation and analgesia acting at the locus ceruleous, resulting in sedation similar to natural sleep. Side effects include hypotension and bradycardia. A recent randomised controlled trial comparing 1 µg/kg intranasal dexmedetomidine and 0.2 µg/kg intranasal midazolam as a premedicant for children undergoing dental procedures showed that although dexmedetomidine had a slower onset of action (20–40 minutes compared to 10–25 minutes), it produced more effective sedation with a better side-effect profile, with significantly less postoperative agitation and no nasal irritation. Both agents had a similar postoperative recovery time, i.e. of 27 minutes [19]. A similar study showed intranasal dexmedetomidine produced superior sedation when compared to oral midazolam [20].

Ketamine acts as an N-methyl-D-aspartate receptor antagonist and nitric oxide synthase inhibitor resulting in analgesia, amnesia and dissociative sedation while maintaining cardiorespiratory function. NICE has produced guidelines into its use for procedural sedation in children, recommending it to be given either intravenously or intramuscularly [21]. Intranasal ketamine has been shown to be an effective analgesic for moderate-to-severe pain in children at doses 0.5–1 mg/kg and has been successfully utilised in prehospital and military settings [22]. A recent systematic review showed that intranasal ketamine is safe with no serious adverse effects and can successfully be used to sedate children for dental and minor surgical procedures with a time to the onset of action ranging between 3.5 and 9.5 minutes [22]. The published studies in this area to date are limited so, although the evidence is promising, there is still a need for further research.

Desmopressin for enuretic and bleeding disorders

Desmopressin is a synthetic analogue of the endogenous pituitary hormone antidiuretic hormone, also known as vasopressin. Its full name is 1-deamino-8-D-arginine vasopressin and so it is often called DDAVP. Desmopressin can be delivered to a child via six different routes; intravenous, intramuscular, subcutaneous, oral tablet, sublingual fast-melting tablet or intranasal spray.

Owing to its antidiuretic effects, desmopressin is the first-line pharmacological treatment option for enuretic disorders such as central diabetes insipidus and nocturnal enuresis. Patients with diabetes insipidus and primary nocturnal enuresis have low night time levels of antidiuretic hormone in their plasma and, therefore, cannot sufficiently concentrate their urine at night, resulting in large volumes of low osmolality urine. Primary nocturnal enuresis is subdivided into monosymptomatic and nonmonosymptomatic depending on whether the child also experiences other symptoms such as increased or decreased frequency of micturition or daytime enuresis. A Cochrane systematic review of response of children with monosymptomatic primary nocturnal enuresis to desmopressin showed that one third of children respond fully to desmopressin, one third show a partial response and the rest do not respond at all [23]. Other contributing factors may explain the variable response to desmopressin, including hyperactive or small bladder volumes, difficulties rousing a child from sleep, obstructive sleep apnoea, or intrinsic renal or electrolyte disturbances.

Intranasal desmopressin was a popular treatment option for enuretic disorders before sublingual fast melts were commercially available, because of ease in administering at home. Even in the group of children with partially responsive primary monosymptomatic nocturnal enuresis, intranasal desmopressin markedly reduces nocturnal urine output as well as sodium urinary excretion [24].

However, the main risk associated with desmopressin is hyponatraemia due to water overload. A systematic literature review published in 2007 compared oral and intranasal desmopressin and showed that intranasal desmopressin was associated with a higher risk of hyponatraemia than the oral formulation, especially in children under the age of 6, potentially due to dosing difficulties [25]. Families are advised to ensure the child does not drink more than normal, including during swimming, to avoid water overload and to stop taking desmopressin when there is a risk of dehydration such as with gastroenteritis.

Desmopressin also causes an increase in endogenous levels of coagulant factors VIII and von Willebrand factor, and has been used to treat von Willebrand's disease and mild to moderate haemophilia A since the 1970s [26].

In the United Kingdom, desmopressin is advocated as first-line treatment for prophylaxis and treatment of bleeding in patients with mild haemophilia A, carriers of haemophilia A and mild von Willebrand's disease to avoid exposure to blood products and factor concentrates [27]. At home, desmopressin can either be given via the subcutaneous or intranasal route. A study from Great Ormond Street showed that, at doses of 150 μg for children under 40 kg in weight and 300 μg for those heavier than 40 kg, intranasal desmopressin was safe and efficacious for children with bleeding disorders [28]. The authors, however, say that at their institution, intranasal desmopressin is not used in children under the age of 3 because of the risk of hyponatraemic-induced seizures.

Desmopressin also causes a rise in endogenous ristocetin cofactor, important in platelet aggregation, and has, therefore, been proposed to be a suitable treatment for congenital disorders of platelet function [26].

Vaccination

Many pathogens causing disease in humans colonise mucosal surfaces. Some vaccines therefore target mucosal surfaces, stimulating local immunity to induce systemic immunity. An example of this is the work being done on producing a vaccine against Group A streptococcus. This streptococcus can infect human hosts via skin or nasal mucosa; a vaccine targeted to the nasal mucosa could stimulate immunoglobulin A (IgA) antibodies to prevent pharyngeal colonisation as well as IgG antibodies to provide systemic immunity, protecting against Group A streptococcal invasion via both cutaneous and mucosal entry sites [29].

An intranasal vaccine that is now available on the UK immunisation schedule is the intranasal live attenuated vaccine against seasonal and pandemic influenza, currently offered to children aged 2–4 years. Because it induces a local mucosal as well as systemic immunity, it confers longer-term protection and better cross-protection than the intramuscular influenza vaccine [30]. The intranasal influenza vaccine is contraindicated in severe asthma or active wheezing, and as it is administered intranasally it can cause some local nasal symptoms, but otherwise has the same adverse effects as the intramuscular influenza vaccine.

Local actions on the nose and upper respiratory tract

Some intranasal medications are used for their local, topical actions in children. A Cochrane systematic review published in 2012 compared evidence for intranasal 0.5% neomycin plus 0.1% chlorhexidine against topical petroleum jelly or surgical cautery for the management of recurrent nosebleeds in children [31]. Five studies were identified involving 468 children but the results were inconclusive. The authors concluded that optimal management of children with recurrent epistaxis was unknown but there is a role for topical intranasal treatments.

Another Cochrane review was published in 2013 looking at the role of intranasal steroids in acute sinusitis in both adults and children [32]. Sinusitis is due to inflammation of nasal mucosa and presents as a prolonged history of 7–10 days of cough, coryza, facial pain and fever. It has been theorised that topical anti-inflammatory treatments would reduce inflammation and, therefore, reduce symptoms. The authors of the review concluded that intranasal corticosteroids improve and alleviate symptoms compared to placebo. Intranasal corticosteroids were not found to be associated with any significant side effects although did cause headache, epistaxis and itching. Although these results may indicate that topical corticosteroids help relieve the symptoms of acute sinusitis, diagnosing acute sinusitis in children can be difficult with a significant proportion of children experiencing resolution of symptoms without any treatment.

With children presenting with viral upper respiratory tract infections placing a significant burden on primary care physicians and emergency departments, an effective treatment for the common cold would be an attractive prospect. The third Cochrane review, published in 2013, looked at the evidence for using intranasal ipratropium bromide to alleviate symptoms of the common cold [33]. The authors reported seven trials involving 2144 children and adults, four of which showed an improvement in global assessment. Although intranasal ipratropium was found to be effective in treating rhinorrhoea, it had no effect on nasal congestion. The evidence is limited and with side effects reported to include nasal dryness, blood-tinged mucous and epistaxis, intranasal ipratropium is unlikely to become a popular treatment in children.

FUTURE APPLICATIONS IN PAEDIATRICS

Research into intranasal medications has by no means reached a plateau. There is ongoing research into introducing gene therapy via the intranasal route [5] tying in with work on the nose to brain theory for centrally acting drugs such as carbamazepine, risperidone and clonazepam [6]. There are publications about work into deoxyribonucleic acid-based vaccines against the viruses such as the severe acute respiratory syndrome coronavirus which could be given via the intranasal route [29]. There is also work underway on modifying drugs to increase contact time with the nasal mucosa. This can be done by adding polymers, gels and polysaccharides to increase absorption and by adding penetration enhancers to allow smaller volumes to be used [5]. And most excitingly perhaps, there is ongoing research to find ways to overcome the difficulties faced with drugs with a large molecular size, which can get caught in the mucous layer and swept posteriorly to be swallowed. This includes medications such as insulin with particular emphasis on preventing diabetes in susceptible children [10].

Intranasal drugs are already part of the here and now, but are likely to play an even bigger role in future pharmaceutical development with exciting treatments on the horizon.

Key points for clinical practice

- Intranasal medications are fast acting because they avoid first-pass metabolism. The ideal characteristic of an intranasal drug is one that is lipophilic at physiological pH with a low molecular weight and high solubility in water.
- Because painful cannulation is avoided, intranasal medications are favoured by parents and are highly acceptable to most children. Many intranasal medications can be administered at home, preventing the need for hospital admission.
- Intranasal diamorphine and fentanyl are recommended for the acute management of severe pain in the paediatric emergency department.
- Intranasal midazolam is more efficacious at terminating active seizure activity than rectal diazepam as time to seizure cessation is shorter with a lower risk of respiratory depression.
- Intranasal midazolam is also effective at producing sedation for painful or frightening procedures, but is not always tolerated well by children because of its low pH. There is emerging evidence that intranasal ketamine and intranasal dexmedetomidine may be viable options for sedation.
- Intranasal sumatriptan is a good treatment modality at managing acute migraine in adolescents.
- Desmopressin can be administered intranasally in mild haemophilia A, von Willebrand's disease and many enuretic disorders but carers should be warned of the risk of hyponatraemia, which may results in hyponatraemic seizures if sodium levels drop very low.
- Intranasal vaccines, such as the influenza vaccine, may be better at preventing infection than parental vaccines.
- There are many intranasal formulations of treatments of local nasal disorders such as epistaxis, sinusitis and the common cold, but the evidence is lacking for their routine use in paediatrics.

REFERENCES

1. Del Pizzo J, Callahan JM. Intranasal medications in paediatric emergency medicine. Pediatr Emerg Care 2014; 30:496–504.
2. Goldman RD. Intranasal drug delivery for children with acute illness. Curr Drug Ther 2006; 1:127–130.
3. Hadley G, Maconochie I, Jackson A. A survey of intranasal medication use in the paediatric emergency setting in England and Wales. Emerg Med J 2010; 27:553–554.
4. Mudd S. Intranasal fentanyl for pain management in children: a systematic review of the literature. J Pediatr Health Care 2011; 25:316–322.
5. Prommer E, Thompson L. Intranasal fentanyl for pain control: current status with a focus on patient considerations. Patient Prefer Adherence 2011; 5:157–164.
6. Suman JD. Current understanding of nasal morphology and physiology as a drug delivery target. Drug Deliv Transl Res 2013; 3:4—15.
7. Wermeling DP. A response to the opioid overdose epidemic: naloxone nasal spray. Drug Deliv Transl Res 2013; 3:63–74.
8. Finn M, Harris D. Intranasal fentanyl for analgesia in the paediatric emergency department. Emerg Med J 2010; 27:300–301.

9. Royal College of Emergency Medicine (RCEM). Management of Pain in Children. RCEM Best Practice Guideline CEM4682. London: RCEM, Revised 2013.

10. Reagan L, Chapman AR, Celnik A, et al. Nose and vein, speed and pain: comparing the use of intranasal diamorphine and intravenous morphine in a Scottish paediatric emergency department. Emerg Med J 2013; 30:49–52.

11. Telfer P, Criddle J, Sandell J, et al. Intranasal diamorphine for acute sickle cell pain. Arch Dis Child 2009; 94:979–980.

12. Yong JWL, Anand G. Does intranasal sumatriptan use relieve migraine in children and young people? Arch Dis Child 2013; 98:82–84.

13. Humphries LK, Eiland LS. Treatment of acute seizures: is intranasal midazolam a viable option? J Pediatr Pharmacol Ther 2013; 18:79–87.

14. O'Regan ME, Brown JK, Clarke M. Nasal rather than rectal benzodiazepines in the management of acute childhood seizures. Dev Med Child Neurol 1996; 38:1037–1045.

15. National Institute for Health and Clinical Excellence (NICE). The epilepsies: the diagnosis and management of the epilepsies in adults and children in primary and secondary care. NICE clinical guideline 137. NICE, 2012.

16. Wilson MT, Macleod S, O'Regan ME. Nasal/buccal midazolam use in the community. Arch Dis Child 2004; 89:50–51.

17. Allan A, Cullen J. Best BETS from the Manchester Royal Infirmary. BET 1: Intranasal lorazepam is an acceptable alternative to intravenous lorazepam in the control of acute seizures in children. Emerg Med J 2013; 30:768–769.

18. Klein EJ, Brown JC, Kobayashi A, et al. A randomised clinical trial comparing oral, aerosolized intranasal and aerosolized buccal midazolam. Ann Emerg Med 2011; 58:323–329.

19. Sheta SA, Al-Sarheed MA, Abdelhalim AA. Intranasal dexmedetomidine vs midazolam for premedication in children undergoing complete dental rehabilitation: a double-blinded randomized controlled trial. Pediatr Anaesth 2014; 24:181–189.

20. Yuen VM, Hui TW, Irwin MG, et al. A comparison of intranasal dexmedetomidine and oral midazolam for premedication in pediatric anesthesia: a double-blinded randomized controlled trial. Anesthesiology 2008; 69:972–975.

21. National Institute of Clinical Excellence (NICE). Sedation in Children and Young People. NICE Clinical Guideline 112 (CG112). London: NICE, 2010.

22. Hall D, Robinson A. Intranasal ketamine for procedural sedation. Emerg Med J 2014; 31:775–791.

23. Glazener CM, Evans JH. Desmopressin for nocturnal enuresis in children. Cochrane Database Syst Rev 2000; 2:CD002112.

24. Kamperis K, Rittig S, Radvanska E, et al. The effect of desmopressin on renal water and solute handling in desmopressin resistant monosymptomatic nocturnal enuresis. J Urol 2008; 180:707–714.

25. Robson WLM, Leung AKC, Norgaard JP. The comparative safety of oral versus intranasal desmopressin for the treatment of children with nocturnal enuresis. J Urol 2007; 178:24–30.

26. Coppola A, Di Minno G. Desmopressin in inherited disorders of platelet function. Haemophilia 2008; 14:31–39.

27. UK Haemophilia Centre Doctors Organisation Guidelines. Guideline on the selection and use of therapeutic products to treat haemophilia and other hereditary bleeding disorders. Haemophilia 2008; 14:671–684.

28. Khair K, Baker K, Mathias M, et al. Intranasal desmopressin (Octim): a safe and efficacious treatment option for children with bleeding disorders. Haemophilia 2007; 13:548–551.

29. Zaman M, Chandrudu S. Strategies for intranasal delivery of vaccines. Drug Deliv Transl Res 2013; 3:100–109.

30. Jefferson T, Rivetti A, Di Pietrantonj C, et al. Vaccines for preventing influenza in healthy children. Cochrane Database Syst Rev 2012; 8:CD004879.

31. Qureishi A, Burton MJ. Interventions for recurrent idiopathic epistaxis (nosebleeds) in children (Review). Cochrane Database Syst Rev 2012, 9:CD004461.

32. Zalmanovici Trestioreanu A, Yaphe J. Intranasal steroids for acute sinusitis. Cochrane Database Syst Rev 2013, 12:CD005149.

33. AlBalawi ZH, Othman SS, AlFaleh K. Intranasal ipratropium bromide for the common cold. Cochrane Database Syst Rev 2015, 6:CD008231.

34. Walsh J, Bickmann D, Breitkreutz J, et al. Delivery devices for the administration of pediatric formulations: overview of current practice, challenges and recent developments. Intl J Pharm 2011; 415:221–231.
35. Simons FE, Gu X, Johnston LM, et al. Can epinephrine inhalations be substituted for epinephrine injection in children at risk from systemic anaphylaxis? Pediatrics 2000; 5:1040–1044.
36. Kundoor V, Dalby RN. Effect of formulation- and administration-related variables on deposition pattern of nasal spray pumps evaluated using a nasal cast. Pharm Res 2011; 28:1895–1904.

Chapter 10

Introducing paediatric life-support courses into a low-income country

Tom Lissauer, Martin Becker, Samuel Van Steirteghem, John Wachira, Lisine Tuyisenge

INTRODUCTION

Paediatric life-support courses are increasingly introduced into low-income countries as a rapid method of training health professionals in the recognition and initial treatment of sick children [1]. This chapter describes the introduction of a paediatric life-support course into Rwanda, the approach adopted and an analysis of what went well and the difficulties encountered. We have also included recommendations which may be useful for others intending to introduce life-support courses into a low-income country. While we are concentrating on paediatric life-support courses, similar issues will arise for other courses as well as teaching and training in low-income countries.

BACKGROUND

Rwanda has a population of 10.5 million and 17% of the population is under 5 years old. In common with many low- and middle-income countries, Rwanda has made determined efforts to achieve the Millennium Development Goal 4 (MDG4) target of reducing mortality of children under five years old between 1990 and 2015 by two thirds. Considerable progress has been made (**Figure 10.1**). In 1990, under five mortality was 151/1000 live births, increasing to 250/1000 after the genocide in 1994, and is anticipated to be one of the few countries to reach its MDG4 target of 50/1000 live births in 2015. This has been achieved in spite of ranking 167/187 on the Human Development Index and having a total health expenditure of $56 per capita in 2010. Many improvements in the organisation of health care delivery have been made, including universal health insurance and a marked

Tom Lissauer MBBChir FRCPCH, Department of Paediatrics, Imperial College Healthcare NHS Trust, London, UK. E-mail: t.lissauer@ imperial.ac.uk (for correspondence)

Martin Becker MD FRCPCH, Department of Paediatrics, Cambridgeshire Community Services NHS Trust, Hinchingbrooke Hospital, Huntingdon, UK

Samuel Van Steirteghem MD, Department of Paediatrics, Ambroise Paré University Hospital, Mons, Belgium

John Wachira MBChB MMed, Gertrude's Department of Paediatrics, Children Hospital, Nairobi, Kenya

Lisine Tuyisenge MD MSc, Department of Paediatrics, Central University Teaching Hospital of Kigali, Kigali, Rwanda

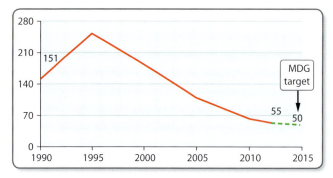

Figure 10.1 Mortality of children under 5 years per 1000 live births in Rwanda since 1990. In 2013, it was 52 per 1000 live births. The Millennium Development Goal 4 (MDG 4) target was 50 per 1000 live births.

increase in nurse-led local health facilities. For children, there has been a high uptake of an extensive immunisation programme (including pneumococcal, haemophilus influenzae type B, rotavirus and second measles vaccines), a marked reduction in mortality from malaria by use of insecticide-treated bed nets and mosquito eradication, an effective programme to prevent the transmission of human immunodeficiency virus (HIV) from mother to child, and the introduction of dedicated ambulances for referral of mothers and children from health facilities to hospitals. There has also been investment in the training of community health workers, who provide early treatment of gastroenteritis with oral rehydration solution and zinc; of malaria (confirmed by rapid diagnostic tests) with artemether–lumefantrine, and acute respiratory infections with amoxicillin. These workers are equipped with mobile phones to call an ambulance and alert health centres or district hospitals [2].

However, mortality in the under-fives remains high, and providing quality healthcare to children admitted to hospital is highly problematic. There are 4 specialist university hospitals, 3 referral, 5 provincial and 33 district hospitals. However, there are <20 paediatricians, and in 2011 there were only 625 doctors, 8273 nurses and 240 midwives in the country [3]. This is fewer than five doctors or nurses per 10,000 population – far less than the 23 doctors and nurses per 10,000 population recommended by the World Health Organization (WHO). There is also no dedicated paediatric nurse training. The assessment and care of sick newborns and children in district hospitals is undertaken by general doctors, often without any specialist or senior paediatric supervision. The initial request for paediatric life-support courses for hospital staff came from the present Minister of Health while one of us (Tom Lissauer) was undertaking a series of training courses in newborn and child health in the country.

CHOICE OF COURSE

As many instructors and lecturers come from high-income countries, they often use the same content for courses as in their home countries. However, many of the diseases encountered, investigations and treatment options available will be different locally. The courses from developed countries are also unlikely to conform to WHO or local guidelines.

We chose to use the Emergency Triage, Assessment and Treatment plus Admission (ETAT+) course. The advantages of this course were:

1. It is designed for hospital health professionals assessing and treating sick children in a hospital setting [4]

2. It covers the 10 most common reasons for sick children to be admitted to hospital in East Africa
3. It is multidisciplinary, with paediatricians, other doctors, nurses and medical officers as participants and instructors
4. It adopts adult learning methods (as in the Advanced Paediatric Life Support and other life-support courses), using case-based scenarios
5. It is an extension of the WHO ETAT course and incorporates the WHO Hospital Care for Sick Children guidelines
6. The instructors are highly trained
7. The course lectures are freely available on the internet [5]
8. The course content is regularly and rigorously updated, with major changes considered using the GRADE (Grading of Recommendations, Assessment, Development and Evaluation) system [6,7]
9. Its development and introduction into hospitals in Kenya has been extensively researched [8]
10. It has a well-developed management structure, under the Kenya Paediatric Association, and has been incorporated into the Kenya Ministry of Health's Operating Plans
11. The Kenya Paediatric Association was willing to assist us by providing instructors for courses in Rwanda.

COURSE CONTENT AND STRUCTURE

The standard course itself is an intensive 5-day course (**Table 10.1**). It consists of lectures (11 hours), demonstrations and practice of practical procedures, case scenarios (22 hours), audit and quality improvement (including reviews of selected patient case notes; 3 hours)

Table 10.1 Topics covered in Emergency Triage, Assessment and Treatment plus Admission course	
Initial assessment	Triage
	Recognition of the sick child
Resuscitation	Neonatal resuscitation
	Cardio-pulmonary resuscitation of children
Clinical conditions	Diarrhoea/dehydration and shock
	Pneumonia
	Asthma
	Malaria
	Malnutrition
	Sepsis/Meningitis
	Convulsions
	Hypoglycaemia
	Neonatal – preterm, sepsis, jaundice, nutrition
Procedures	Oxygen, intraosseous needle insertion, lumbar puncture
	Prescribing

and a final assessment, personal feedback and presentation of certificates (4 hours). About one and a half days are devoted to care of newborn infants.

In order to pass the course,, candidates have to achieve a predetermined pass mark for a knowledge test and pass the clinical skills scenarios. If achieved, a certificate is awarded.

ESTABLISHING THE PROJECT

An Imperial College–Rwanda health partnership was formed, between Imperial College Healthcare NHS Trust and the Rwanda Paediatric Association and the National University of Rwanda (now University of Rwanda, College of Medicine and Health Sciences) and Ministry of Health in Rwanda. The aim was to improve the recognition and management of sick newborn infants and children in hospital using the ETAT+ course. This involved (**Figure 10.2**):

1. Establishing acceptance of the course in Rwanda
2. Training all the medical students for two academic years (six courses)
3. Running the course in six district hospitals
4. Establishing a group of local instructors
5. Creating the local infrastructure for continuation of the course

A grant was obtained from the International Health Partnership Funding Scheme (Imperial College–Rwanda Health Partnership; principal investigator and co-ordinator in United Kingdom, Dr Tom Lissauer and in Rwanda, Dr Lisine Tuyisenge, administered by THET for UK Aid). An endorsement by the Ministry of Health in Rwanda was crucial for the introduction of the course.

GAINING COURSE ACCEPTANCE

As the course and its method of training was new to Rwanda, we needed to gain the support of senior medical staff within paediatrics and allied specialities, e.g. anaesthetics. Therefore we held a 3-day workshop covering all aspects of the course including participation in

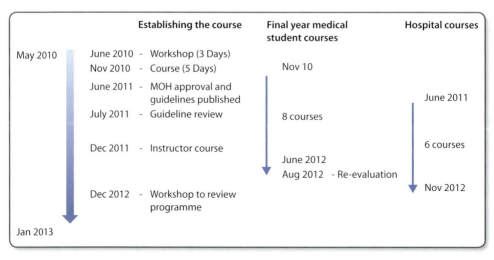

Figure 10.2 Overview of the programme. MOH, Ministry of Health, Rwanda.

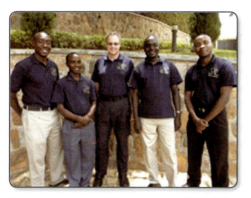

Figure 10.3 Instructors from Kenya who delivered the first Emergency Triage, Assessment and Treatment plus Admission (ETAT+) course in Rwanda.

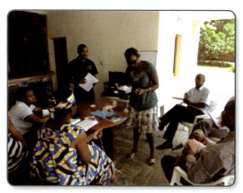

Figure 10.4 Scenario-based teaching using mannikins.

scenario-based teaching (**Figures 10.3** and **10.4**) but excluding the assessment. Time was allowed for participants to go through the course content and identify the need for any local adaptation. This was overseen by a senior paediatrician from the United Kingdom.

Fortunately, the course was enthusiastically received. A further full course and content review was required to attract and accommodate all key senior staff. A final review of the course was undertaken at a workshop conducted by the Rwanda Paediatric Association. Very few amendments were required and acceptance of the course enabled us to obtain endorsement by the Ministry of Health. An official guideline booklet was produced and printed. This process meant that paediatricians were conversant with the ETAT+ approach and guidelines. It also allowed us to overcome some initial scepticism about having nursing and medical officer as instructors for medical staff, and it enabled us to start identifying potential instructors.

MEDICAL STUDENT COURSES

All final-year medical students were enrolled during two academic years. Courses were conducted by Kenyan instructors in English, which had recently been adopted as the language of tuition for medicine, replacing French. This was a major advantage, as few of the Kenyan instructors spoke any French. The medical students were keen to participate and rapidly learnt how to conduct scenario-based teaching. The same course was applied as used for hospital staff, including the same final knowledge and clinical skills assessment. Altogether, eight medical student courses were held over two academic years; 217 medical students and some graduate trainees and nurses completed the course. The pass rate was 97%.

LOCAL INSTRUCTORS

When a sufficient number of potential local instructors had been identified, an instructor training course was held. The course provided generic instructor training and was conducted by experienced Kenyan instructors; 24 new from Rwanda and four from Uganda were trained (**Figure 10.5**). To complete the instructor training, participants acted as an

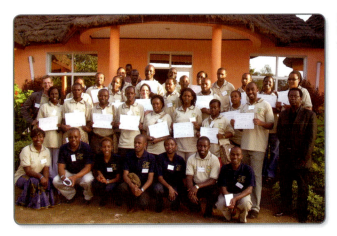

Figure 10.5 First cohort of new Rwandan instructors and the Kenyan trainers.

instructor on two courses under the supervision of experienced instructors, and then worked alongside a trained instructor for two further courses. This intensive training of instructors was adapted from the high-quality training of European Resuscitation Council instructors.

HOSPITAL COURSES

 Courses were conducted in six district hospitals in different parts of the country. Initially, the course was conducted in English with a health professional available to translate into French as required. Course material was also available in French. However, as many of the staff in the district hospitals spoke only French, this approach was not optimal, especially for the scenario-based sessions and assessment. Courses were subsequently conducted in French or Kinyarwanda by Rwandan instructors. A Kenyan instructor overseeing the course, led the daily instructor briefing and debriefing and provided performance feedback and mentorship for instructors.

At the six district hospitals, 177 health professionals completed the course, with a pass rate of 80%.

EVALUATION

Medical student course re-evaluation

At the end of the academic year in 2012, we re-evaluated of the medical students who had attended ETAT+ courses during that academic year [9]. Attendance was voluntary, but it provided students an opportunity to refresh their knowledge and skills and receive personal feedback of their performance. This allowed us to compare their knowledge test results before and after the course and at re-evaluation. We also compared clinical skills performance after the course and at re-evaluation. The clinical skills scenarios were neonatal resuscitation and the management of an acutely sick child with shock from dehydration. Performance was marked according to standardised criteria. To pass the skills assessment, candidates had to pass both scenarios; if all standardised criteria were not met in one scenario, candidates were given feedback and were allowed to retake. If a

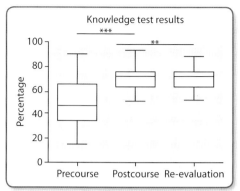

Figure 10.6 Knowledge test results showing the percentage of correct answers. Lines show median percentage, boxes demonstrate inter-quartile range and whiskers show maximum and minimum results. ***, $P < 0.0001$, **, $P > 0.1$ by Wilcoxon matched-pairs signed rank test. Reproduced with permission from Tuyisenge L, Kyamanya P, Van Seierteghem S, et al. Knowledge and skills retention following Emergency triage, assessment and treatment plus admission course for final year medical students in Rwanda: a longitudinal cohort study. Arch Dis Child 2014; 99:11993–11997.

student did not reach the required standard after a retake, or if they failed both scenarios at their first attempt, they were judged to have failed and were not allowed to retake the scenarios.

Re-evaluation was attended by 84 of the 88 students had who completed four courses (**Figure 10. 6**). Knowledge tests taken before and after the course showed significant improvement, from a median 47% (interquartile range 35–65) of correct answers to 71% (interquartile range 63–75) ($P < 0.0001$). On retesting 3–9 months later, the results were similar to postcourse at 67% (interquartile range 52–75, $P > 0.1$).

For the two clinical skills scenarios, immediately after completion of the course, 98% passed both scenarios, 38% after a retake and 2% failed both scenarios. At re-evaluation 74% passed with 30% requiring a retake, 18% failed both scenarios and a further 8% failed after retake, a significant deterioration ($P < 0.0001$).

This re-evaluation showed that almost all the students performed well on knowledge and skills immediately after the course. Knowledge was maintained 3–9 months later, although this was likely to have been augmented by the students sitting their final examinations shortly beforehand. Clinical skills declined, which is in keeping with the results of follow-up studies after other life-support courses, both for junior and senior health professionals. However, passing the clinical skills scenarios required detailed sequential steps to be performed, and most of the medical students were able to perform them satisfactorily after feedback, suggesting that they had retained the concepts but needed reminding of the details. In addition, many of the reasons for failing were not checking for signs such as muscle tone and patient colour which are likely to be recognised in real life but needed to be enunciated for a manikin. In addition, failure to follow the exact sequence specified in a rigidly structured assessment may not necessarily result in worse outcomes in clinical practice.

Comparing the time interval in months with performance postcourse and re-evaluation, there was no statistical difference in scores for either the knowledge test or clinical skills scenarios.

Feedback after the courses was obtained by anonymous questionnaires. They showed:
- Clinical scenarios were the most highly rated aspect (80% highly satisfied, 18% satisfied)
- Lectures were also rated highly (59% highly satisfied, 37% satisfied)
- Session on quality improvement involving an audit of the hospital was least highly rated, probably because the students were keener to acquire new knowledge and skills
- Most commented on the excellence of the instructors.

Suggested improvements were:
- The course should be split into two or more sessions to allow more time for clinical scenarios and practical skills
- Avoid information overload
- Add a session on HIV infection.

Hospital courses

Organisation of the hospital courses improved with experience. Initially, hospital staff were often only informed about the course shortly before the start of the course, usually because of a delay in authorisation. In addition, hospital rotas had to be reorganised to allow staff to be available for 5 days, which was difficult as there are a very few staff on the paediatric wards in district hospitals. It was particularly difficult for doctors to attend as they were often covering multiple services. Some staff attending the course were found to have been on call overnight until this issue was raised in advance with hospital directors when course arrangements were made. Getting a significant percentage of key staff to attend was therefore problematic.

Staff were often unable to do precourse preparation making assimilation of the large amount of information more difficult. This was exacerbated by some staff having limited English language skills. For almost all staff, this was their first encounter with scenario-based teaching instead of the traditional, formal lecturing to which they are accustomed, and it took time for them to understand the method and gain enough confidence to participate. For many, it was also their first encounter with multidisciplinary training. Worries about the formal assessment at the end of the course necessitated considerable practice and reassurance. However, feedback from questionnaires after the course showed great appreciation of this style of training and of the high quality of the instructors, but many stated that they would have preferred more time to cover the material.

ADMINISTRATION AND FINANCE

No administrative support was available within the grant, which was problematic as the administrative burden was very considerable. Basic neonatal and child mannikins were brought from the United Kingdom. Toolboxes with items required for demonstrating practical procedures were assembled locally. Lectures and multiple choice questions were also available in French. Hospitals selected to conduct courses were visited in advance to explain the aims of the course and plan logistics with the medical and nursing directors. Venues for the courses had to be identified and organised, as none of the hospitals nor the university were able to provide on-site accommodation. Off-site venues were preferred to avoid staff being called away to deal with day-to-day problems.

Space was required not only to conduct lectures but also for the small group teaching and case-based scenarios. Courses were planned for up to 32 candidates, with 5 instructors and case-scenario teaching in 4 groups of up to 8 candidates. We brought neonatal and child mannikins and everything needed to ensure that the course ran smoothly including projectors, extension cables, etc. Beverages and lunch were provided on site to allow the course to keep to a strict timetable. Accommodation and travel for Kenyan instructors had to be organised. This placed a heavy administrative load on the project coordinators, especially as no administrative support existed within the Rwanda Paediatric Association.

Finance was difficult as we ran on a very tight budget and encountered many unanticipated extra costs. Examples were the university changing from three to four residency programmes per year, which required us to provide two additional courses to train all the medical students. We also had to provide an additional introductory course and workshop to gain clinician's acceptance of the project. We initially provided photocopied handouts of course content but subsequently provided this and a range of associated material on memory sticks, together with pocket-sized booklets of the guidelines. We did not have to pay for using the ETAT+ course material.

Many administrative obstacles had to be overcome, especially as the Rwanda Paediatric Association had no working capital, yet most venues required deposits to be paid in advance. We were fortunate that a Belgian paediatrician based in Rwanda (Samuel Van Steirteghem) obtained some additional funding from the Belgian Technical Co-operation, otherwise we would have had to scale back our programme.

POSSIBLE COURSE MODIFICATIONS

With the current 5-day course, candidates and instructors set aside a specific time period for a comprehensive course, and after passing the assessment, candidates are 'ETAT+ trained'. An advantage of a 5-day course is that it takes some time for candidates to get used to the style of training, particularly the scenario-based teaching.

An alternative would be to run several short courses. This would avoid information overload and allow reinforcement of key information and case scenarios. The course could be divided into separate components, e.g. newborn and children. Health professionals only looking after newborn infants would not need to attend training about children and those looking after children would need to cover only essential aspects of newborn care, e.g. newborn resuscitation. However, this requires more administration and travelling for instructors, and certainly would have been problematic for us with instructors coming from Kenya. Getting approval for time off to attend several ETAT+ training sessions may prove to be more difficult than a single longer course.

The course could be shortened by requiring candidates to read the lecture material beforehand. Whereas medical students had their own laptops and computers are available in the university, this may be more problematic for staff in district hospitals. The course could be enhanced by e-learning materials (which are being produced), and participants could be sent reminders and learning materials on mobile electronic devices. All these changes would need to be evaluated.

SUSTAINABILITY

To scale up the programme to provide training for all health professionals caring for sick children in hospitals, numerous courses would need to be conducted.

We have shown that medical students can master the course content and achieve a high pass rate, and are able to retain knowledge and skills in spite of their limited clinical experience. We advocate this as a useful way of introducing the ETAT+ approach to medical staff. In Rwanda, this will require four or more courses per year as the medical school intake is increasing and will need to be undertaken by the university in the future.

We estimate that 30 courses would be required to train most hospital staff in Rwanda, followed by five courses a year to allow for staff turnover.

Ongoing training for all staff needs to be provided to maintain knowledge and skills, with both regular on-site refresher sessions and staff retaking the course periodically.

New instructors need to be trained and must be able and prepared to devote time to conducting courses regularly to maintain their skills.

Organising these programmes requires leadership, currently provided by the Rwanda Paediatric Association and Ministry of Health. It also requires finance, a major issue when external funding is no longer available. This will need to be obtained either from participants or from the Ministry of Health. One also needs to consider the controversial issue of 'per diems', widely expected for attendance and travel to courses for both participants and instructors.

The course itself needs to be developed and updated. The willingness of the Kenya Paediatric Association to allow the course to be adopted in Rwanda, to arrange for their highly trained instructors to conduct courses and to allow Rwandan health professionals to participate in the course development, has been of enormous benefit in establishing the course in Rwanda. Running courses with similar structure and content throughout East Africa is highly desirable, but finances will need to be put in place for this to be maintained.

This description has focussed on establishing a structured programme for training hospital staff in the recognition and management of sick children. Implementing ETAT+ courses has been used in Kenya to spearhead improvements in clinical practice and care in hospitals [8], and we conducted a number of quality improvement projects at the hospitals where courses were conducted. In several hospitals, the course and quality improvement programmes were followed by structural improvements in the paediatric department, including new assessment areas for admission of sick children, the enlargement of neonatal units and the introduction of kangaroo mother care for preterm infants.

The project's sustainability has been enhanced by a subsequent ETAT+ course programme in Rwanda, Kenya and Uganda under the auspices of the Royal College of Paediatrics and Child Health, which provides further courses for medical students, hospital health professionals and instructor training. A number of courses have also been sponsored by other non-governmental organisations.

CONCLUSION

This project was the first step in establishing the ETAT+ course in Rwanda.
Many health professionals and non-governmental organisations rush into low-income countries and conduct one or a few courses and then leave. We have adopted a very different approach in order to create a course which has been adopted nationally and aims to become sustainable.

Key points for clinical practice

- A suitable course needs to be identified or adapted for local conditions. It needs to have the infrastructure to be regularly updated using evidence-based methodology.
- Key senior health professionals need to be identified and become fully acquainted with the course content for its guidelines to be endorsed nationally and adopted by the Ministry of Health. This is also essential in order to get the guidelines incorporated into clinical practice and training.

- Delivering the course to final-year medical students enables all new doctors to be trained and be familiar with the guidelines, including those in other specialties who treat children but would be unlikely to attend a course dedicated to paediatric practice. We have shown that, in spite of their limited paediatric clinical experience, medical students were able to perform well and pass the course, and their knowledge and skills were well maintained when re-evaluated 3–9 months later.

- The high-quality of instructors is paramount. Crucial to the success of this programme was the excellence of the clinical instructors, whose professionalism was repeatedly commended. Potential instructors had been identified from their high level of performance not only in assessment of knowledge but also during training and assessment of clinical skills. They then underwent generic instructor training followed by supervised performance as instructors with mentorship and assessment. This is in contrast to the cascade strategy often adopted to train large numbers in low-income countries, where a group of master trainers are appointed, receive course training and teaching materials, and this process is repeated until all health workers have received training.

- A programme of regular refresher sessions is required but has to be well organised and maintained; we have found this needs to be done by ETAT+ instructors to be successful.

- The course has been strengthened by its regional identity for East Africa. An advantage is that staff coming from other East African countries will have received similar training. Rwandan paediatricians are now involved in evidence-based workshops conducted in Kenya and attend conferences and other educational activities in East Africa.

- Although initially organised from overseas, the course now has local ownership both in its organisation and provision.

- The foundations have been laid for a sustainable programme of courses but considerable leadership, finance and vision will be required to scale up the programme to train all health professionals caring for sick children in hospital and for their training to be maintained.

REFERENCES

1. Ralston ME, Day LT, Slusher TM, et al. Global paediatric advanced life support: improving child survival in limited resource settings. Lancet 2013; 381:256 – 265.
2. Mugeni C, Levine AC, Munyaneza RM, et al. Nationwide implementation of integrated community case management of childhood illness in Rwanda. Glob Health Sci Pract 2014; 2:328–341.
3. Binagwaho A, Kyamanywa P, Farmer P, et al. The human resources for health program in Rwanda – a new Partnership. N Engl J Med 2013; 369: 2054–2059.
4. English M, Wamae A, Nyamai R, et al. Implementing locally appropriate guidelines and training to improve care of serious illness in Kenyan hospitals—A story of scaling-up (and down and left and right). Arch Dis Child 2011; 96:285–290.
5. ETAT+ (Emergency Triage Assessment and Treatment plus Admission Care) www.idoc-africa.org. (Last accessed May 2015).
6. Irimu G, Wamae A, Wasunna A, et al. Developing and introducing evidence based clinical practice guidelines for serious illness in Kenya. Arch Dis Child 2008; 93:799–804.
7. English M, Opiyo N. Getting to grips with GRADE – perspective from a low-income setting. J Clin Epidemiol 2011; 64:708–710.
8. Ayieko P, Ntoburi S, Wagai J, et al. A Multifaceted Intervention to Implement Guidelines and Improve Admission Paediatric Care in Kenyan District Hospitals: a Cluster Randomised Trial. PLoS Med 2011; 8:e1001018.
9. Tuyisenge L, Kyamanya P, Van Seierteghem S, et al. Knowledge and skills retention following Emergency Triage, Assessment and Treatment plus Admission course for final year medical students in Rwanda: a longitudinal cohort study. Arch Dis Child 2014; 99:11993–11997.

Chapter 11

Rehabilitation after acquired brain injury in childhood

Hayley Griffin, Robert Forsyth

BACKGROUND

Definitions

An acquired brain injury (ABI) is any insult to the brain acquired after the perinatal period and causing impairment to function, or with the potential to cause impairment. Conditions such as meningitis/encephalitis, cardiac arrest and profound hypotension cause ABI among others. The term 'acquired brain injury' includes traumatic brain injury (TBI).

A TBI is any forceful insult by the transfer of kinetic energy to the brain, either accidental or nonaccidental, e.g. following a road traffic collision, a fall, or other nonaccidental injury.

The severity of brain injury has historically been notoriously difficult to define. Many different criteria, including the time to recovery of awareness, length of amnesia, length of time to first follow commands, have all been used. There are many approaches to determining severity in the literature, but none are entirely satisfactory.

In this chapter, we will define the severity of brain injury using the Glasgow Coma Scale (GCS) score. Severe brain injury can be considered GCS 8 or less, moderate with GCS 9–12 and mild with GCS 13 or greater. It is generally accepted that GCS is unreliable in determining severity of injury, particularly, in younger children, so this classification is not ideal. The most useful component of the GCS is the motor scale, and a recently published study [1] concluded that the motor score alone can be just as useful as all scores combined, being predictive of severe TBI. The relative unreliability of the verbal and eye components may be for a number of reasons, including difficulty in obtaining the co-operation of a frightened and injured child.

Prevalence

Traumatic brain injury accounts for 3.4% of emergency department attendances of children under the age of 16. It accounts for 15–20% deaths in young people between the ages of 15 and 25. Head injury is the most common cause of death and disability in people aged 1– 40 years in the United Kingdom.

Hayley Griffin MBBS BSc MRCPCH, Child Development Centre, Nottingham Children's Hospital, UK. Email: hayleygriffin@doctors.org. uk (for correspondence)

Robert Forsyth FRCPCH DCH PhD BMBCh MA(Cantab), Institute of Neuroscience, Royal Victoria Hospital, Newcastle, UK

Despite this, the incidence of death from TBI is low, at around 0.2% of those who present to the emergency department. However, the incidence of hospitalisation of children under the age of 16 with TBI in England ranges from 280 to 500 per 100,000 per year. Of these, approximately 6% will have sustained a severe brain injury, 8% a moderate brain injury and 86% a mild brain injury. Although the rates of early morbidity and early motor morbidity in particular are lower in children with mild brain injuries than those with more severe injuries, the longer-term behavioural and cognitive consequences of mild TBI contribute to a larger overall burden of injury in terms of numbers.

The incidence of ABI, not including TBI, is lower than 6 children per 100,000 per year. In the UK population of 12.4 million children under the age of 16 (Office of National Statistics 2012), this represents 744 children per year who acquire a brain injury secondary to a nontraumatic process. This group comprises children with a range of underlying causes, including infection (meningitis and encephalitis), stroke and brain tumours. The true incidence may be higher than this in reality, but it is not known due to under-reporting.

Epidemiology

The most common cause of head injury in children and young people is as a result of a fall. The most common cause of moderate and severe head injuries in children is related to road traffic collisions [2].

It is estimated that, among children under the age of 2, 64% of all head injuries (excluding uncomplicated skull fractures) are nonaccidental and 95% of serious head injuries are nonaccidental [3]. However, in the context of child abuse as a whole, brain injury occurs in 0.5% of cases.

Risk factors

Traumatic brain injury is associated with a number of risk factors that are discussed below:
1. **Gender.** Boys are 1.4 times more likely to sustain a TBI under the age of 10 years than girls. This increases to 2.2 above the age of 10 [4]
2. **Social deprivation** is associated with a higher incidence of TBI
3. **Pre-existing neurodevelopmental disorders** such as attention deficit hyperactivity disorder (ADHD) can increase risk-taking behaviour, hence increase the risk of TBI

NEUROANATOMY

The effects of brain injury can be divided into two phases:
1. **Primary brain injury** – sustained at the time of the incident. This remains unchanged by early management
2. **Secondary brain injury** – evolves and matures after the primary brain injury and can be caused by raised intracranial pressure and the effects of swelling, amongst other poorly understood secondary neurometabolic cascades. This can lead to reduced oxygenation of the brain tissue and ischaemic damage

Early intervention is aimed at minimising this damage and consists of careful attention to airway, breathing and circulation in resuscitation and ongoing head injury care in the paediatric intensive care unit. However, even with optimal treatment, neurometabolic factors can lead to secondary damage.

After injury, the metabolic demands of the brain increase and the brain enters a phase of 'metabolic crisis'. This leads to increased glucose utilisation and mitochondrial dysfunction in the early stages of injury. In turn, this cascade can lead to chronic cell death, dysfunction and neurodegeneration [5], which contribute to the longer-term morbidity following brain injury. These processes are independent of early care.

In the immature brain, recovery from injury is a complex interplay between recovery and forward progress with developmental processes, which means that children tend to 'grow into' their brain injury, showing cognitive and behavioural difficulties at a later developmental stage than the time of the initial injury. The younger the age at which brain injury occurred, the worse the outcome [6].

The pattern of brain injury may also be an important factor as it may have prognostic implications. The presence of diffuse axonal injury, usually secondary to a high-velocity shearing force, tends to disrupt connections between various cortical and subcortical areas and can lead to disruption of complex brain networks. Children who have suffered a diffuse axonal injury may have deficits similar to those with frontal lobe dysfunction, including difficulties with social and emotional behaviour and cognition. These difficulties may only be identified months or years after the initial injury. This pattern of difficulties in diffuse axonal injury has been found to be independent of the presence of frontal parenchymal lesions [7].

When there is a hypoxic-ischaemic injury to the brain, children tend to have worse outcomes, including a slower and less complete recovery [8].

Children suffering moderate-to-severe TBI have smaller overall brain volumes than their peers following injury. Studies have shown volume loss in selected brain regions including the hippocampus, amygdala, globus pallidus, thalamus, periventricular white matter, cerebellum and brain stem. After injury, children are also more likely to have increased cerebrospinal fluid and ventricular volume. Imaging studies have demonstrated these changes as early as 18 months after injury and independent of atrophy caused by focal lesions [9]. Studies using diffusion tensor imaging have also shown evidence of white matter changes and changes to the corpus callosum following TBI [10].

The hippocampus is also particularly vulnerable to hypoxic damage. If a TBI becomes complicated by raised intracranial pressure, there is a disproportionate decrease in hippocampal growth 5 years after the injury was sustained. This tends to be most noticeable on the ipsilateral side to the impact [11].

EARLY CONSEQUENCES OF ABI

The consequences of ABI and, therefore, the rehabilitation focus can be divided into early, medium and longer term. The acute rehabilitative phase takes place alongside acute neurological or neurosurgical treatment. The second stage should take place in a specialist neurorehabilitation facility and begin after the acute illness phase has ended. The long-term rehabilitation should then be facilitated by the community disability team [12]. There should be seamless progression between the different phases of the rehabilitation journey.

Evidence of the effectiveness and cost benefits of early rehabilitation following brain injury is increasing [13]. It is important that the avoidance of secondary complications is at the forefront of early rehabilitation and any rehabilitation service should aim to meet the psychological needs of children and families during their hospital stay and after discharge from hospital.

In the early stages of the process, the assessment and management of rehabilitation needs may be based around the minimally conscious child and needs to include consideration of the following:

1. Dysautonomia
2. Spasticity and dystonia
3. Swallowing difficulties
4. Post-traumatic epilepsy
5. Bladder, bowel and cardiovascular issues
6. Sleep disorders
7. Sensory disturbances
8. Pain
9. Family disturbance

It is not within the scope of this chapter to discuss the assessment and management of the above complications in detail, but it is important to consider early and expectant management of recognised complications and to ensure that rehabilitation commences early after injury to ensure that these issues are not overlooked. In general, the management of spasticity, dystonia, epilepsy and dysphagia is similar in principle to how these complications are managed in children with cerebral palsy.

Dysautonomia is a concept more specific to ABI and we shall consider this separately. It can be seen in up to 13% of children with brain injury but it is less common in TBI (10%) than hypoxic brain injury after cardiac arrest (31%) [14]. Dysautonomia may comprise a combination of fever, tachypnoea, tachycardia, hypertension, diaphoresis (sweating) and dystonia, and is associated with poorer outcomes after brain injury. The pathophysiology is not well understood, but it is thought to be a result of disinhibition of diencephalic autonomic centres and oversensitivity to nociceptive sensory stimuli.

Management of dysautonomia is mainly symptom control. This can be done through manipulation of the environment including low noise, lights and stimulation and through pharmacological agents such as benzodiazepines, baclofen, clonidine and beta-blockers, amongst others.

LATER CONSEQUENCES OF ABI

A study looking at the educational, vocational and psychosocial outcomes in young adults who had survived a TBI in childhood noted that TBI is a lifelong condition often with delayed presentation of complications [15].

Increasingly, it is being recognised that ABI should be considered a chronic disease, alongside conditions such as diabetes and cystic fibrosis. The cognitive effects of an ABI occurring in early life may only become apparent as the child's developmental trajectory of higher cognitive abilities deviates from that of his/her peer group in later childhood. It is for this reason that academic or social difficulties in a child who has sustained a brain injury in the past should be considered as a potential consequence of the brain injury.

Moderate and severe ABI sustained in infancy or early childhood are associated with more severe and persistent defects. It is important to remember that the effect is on the child's emerging skills rather than an adult's established skills [16]. This means that children who have not had a chance to develop skills, which may normally be expected to emerge later in childhood, may have difficulties acquiring these skills where neural networks are disrupted by early brain injury.

Cognitive manifestations

Studies have shown that children who have suffered a brain injury have poorer executive functioning with less impulse control and poorer problem solving abilities than a control group. Executive function can be described as the ability to plan and solve a problem. Intact executive function is essential to independent adult functioning. Children who fail to develop executive functioning as a result of brain injury are often able to carry out individual components of a task, but do not necessarily have the skills to perform a sequence of events required to complete a more complex task. Intact executive functioning is essential to independent adult living. A child may have the motor ability to carry out individual tasks, such as walking and talking, but the importance of executive function is the ability to integrate and plan tasks to complete a more complex activity, which may consist of a series of smaller tasks.

Following ABI, children's thinking is often rigid and inflexible, and attention control may be poor [17]. There can also be effects on the acquisition of new knowledge owing to impaired declarative learning, with particular effects on acquisition of skills underlying moral reasoning, social cognition and executive functions. Even in mild TBI, children have been shown to have memory difficulties for new information for up to 3 months postinjury.

Complex attention skills (e.g. shifting, divided attention and attentional control) are more vulnerable following TBI and slower to recover than simple attention controls [17]. This has implications for the rehabilitation process, particularly where a child is returning to school and expectations may mismatch his/her abilities. This may be addressed through graduated return to school and less expectation upon tasks such as homework, with adequate rest periods through the school day. Specific techniques such as 'cueing' where a partial cue is provided to assist recall may be helpful.

The challenge for education services is that children in this group have a unique and unusual pattern of learning needs. The so-called 'sleeper effect' means that these learning needs are often difficult to predict at the time of injury and that difficulties may not be apparent until later in development.

Social manifestations

It has been shown that children who have sustained severe brain injury score poorly in tasks related to emotional perception, which is an integral part of social communication. A study of young adults who had sustained severe TBI in their childhood found that they had difficulty in the recognition and interpretation of facial and prosodic emotional cues when compared to a control group of young adults who had suffered mild-to-moderate brain injury in their childhood [18]. Following head injury, a child's social development may be adversely affected; often they lose friends owing to deficits in responding to social cues. Intervention based on pragmatic approaches to make the child aware of behavioural interaction is a logical step to overcome the social isolation that frequently occurs.

It has also been found that people who have suffered a TBI in childhood are overrepresented in the prison population. It is possible that up to 60% of the prison population have suffered significant TBI during childhood. A study from Finland showed that a TBI in childhood or adolescence led to a fourfold relative risk of offending behaviour. This study controlled other factors such as socioeconomic deprivation and family circumstances [19]. The difficulty with this type of study is the effect of recall bias upon results.

Emotional manifestations

Children who have suffered TBI tend to have lower self-esteem than a control sample of their peer group or compared to population norms. This can lead to problems with anxiety and depression and parental stress. Low self-esteem may also adversely affect academic performance and lead to further psychosocial problems. Assessment of psychological effects of brain injury should be made at the time of injury or early in the rehabilitation process and appropriate support should be provided as part of the rehabilitation and reintegration process [20].

Vision/hearing

It is important to consider the effects of ABI on a child's vision and hearing, and ensure that these sensory modalities are tested before the child leaves hospital in cases of moderate and severe ABI. In ABI, cortical visual impairment may be overlooked and may have a considerable impact on morbidity following brain injury.

Likewise, it is important to ensure that hearing is tested. In specific cases of hearing loss, such as ABI secondary to pneumococcal meningitis, there is a short window of opportunity for considering cochlear implant as this is not an option once the cochlear has ossified.

Rehabilitation

This has been defined as a goal-based process which reduces the impact of long-term disabling conditions on daily life [12]. There is increasing evidence for the shorter-term benefits, albeit the evidence for long-term effects is much less clear. Instinctively, it is logical that neurorehabilitation should produce better functional and cognitive longer-term outcomes.

Of utmost importance in the ongoing care of a child with ABI is providing seamless, integrated multidisciplinary care directed towards the needs of the individual child. Co-ordinated team working towards a common set of goals is shown to enhance participation of the child.

The International Classification of Functioning, Disability and Health framework [21] helps us to direct approaches to rehabilitation and care. The simple diagram in **Figure 11.1** shows how the child within his/her environment should be considered, as well as the environment in the context of the child.

Goal-directed approach

A multidisciplinary approach to individual goal setting in rehabilitation is important, with professionals working with the child and family towards common goals. Family satisfaction with this approach is high. Regular team meetings help to assess progress towards goals [22] and show that a unified way of working can be very successful.

Physical considerations

There are a number of medical complications that should be considered during active rehabilitation following the acute phase after ABI. These may include the following:

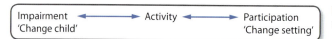

Figure 11.1 Interaction of child and environmental factors.

1. **Spasticity management**, including the prevention of contractures, consideration of botulinum toxin therapy or other pharmacological strategies
2. **Postural support** to ensure optimal positioning through wheelchair support and to prevent complications such as scoliosis
3. **Mobility to optimise independence.** Where possible, this should include weight bearing to minimise the risk of orthopaedic complications such as hip subluxation
4. **Support with care**, e.g. ensuring safe and acceptable methods of feeding, ensuring adequate toilet access or bladder and bowel care, and encouraging independence, where possible, with activities of daily living (appropriate to developmental age)
5. **Developing a communication strategy** and ensuring adequate time to enable processing of language when there may be specific difficulties in this area. This may include rehabilitation of speech or introduction of complex communication aids. Other methods, such as eye pointing or Picture Exchange Communication System (PECS), may also be considered
6. **Sleep**. Children may suffer sleep disturbance for a number of reasons, not least because their circadian rhythm is disrupted by hospitalisation and possibly a stay on the intensive care unit. Supporting a healthy day and night normality with structured bedtime, waking up time and rest times during the day would be the first line of management. Medication such as melatonin may be required to 'reset' the circadian rhythm. Sedatives should be avoided wherever possible as they may cause confusion or resistance to a more structured approach to the bedtime routine

Inpatient rehabilitation approaches

It is important that in the early stages of rehabilitation, environmental factors are adapted to help recovery. Children recovering from moderate and severe ABI have periods of lucidity and periods of confusion. It is, therefore, important that they are nursed within a consistent and calm environment wherever possible with familiar family members and objects.

As the rehabilitation process continues, ensuring a structured timetable of 'normality' is important with timetabled therapy sessions, hospital, school and rest. Visual timetables can be useful as children may have difficulties in memory or language processing. Involving the family in developing a programme of care is beneficial in encouraging recovery.

Discharge planning

Rehabilitation involves frequent assessment of goal attainment or obstacles to achieving goals. It is important when discharge from the inpatient rehabilitation setting is considered that discharge planning is commenced early on and is a flexible process.

Discharge planning meetings allow therapy, education and medical professionals currently involved with the child as an inpatient to identify what needs to be in place for safe and seamless transition to home. These also allow the team taking over the care of the child and the family in the community setting, to better understand the ongoing needs of the child and family.

The child and family should remain central to the discharge planning process. Goal setting should be undertaken keeping a discharge date in mind to ensure that there is adequate provision of services, equipment and expertise in the home and school environment to which the child will return.

LOOKING TO THE FUTURE

Transition to home from the rehabilitation setting can often be a worrying and stressful time for children with ABI and their families. The family should feel supported around this time of transition. This means that adequate preparations have taken place to ensure smooth transition. It is important to consider different settings in which the child will participate upon leaving hospital in order to ensure that participation is maximised.

'Team around the child' meetings

A keyworker should be identified for the family to provide emotional and practical support once the child is discharged. This person provides continuity between the inpatient and community setting where possible.

In children with ongoing complex needs following discharge from hospital, a lead professional, such as a community paediatrician, should be identified to co-ordinate ongoing care and to liaise with education and social care in providing adequate support to the child and family. It is helpful to have regular inter-agency 'Team around the Child' meetings, particularly in the early stages after discharge where the child's needs may be rapidly changing or evolving.

Reintegration into school

As children spend a significant proportion of their lives in the school setting, it is very important that they are involved in reintegration into school from an early stage. Regardless of the severity of brain injury, information sharing with school is key as the cognitive and academic sequelae of ABI are often the most difficult to identify. There may also be little appreciation that academic difficulties may be secondary to brain injury as these can be a 'hidden disability'.

It is possible that following brain injury, the complexity of a child's ongoing needs is such that adaptation of a mainstream school or consideration of a special school placement needs to be discussed. Some children will require additional funding to meet their new needs through an education, health and care plan (which has replaced the statement of special educational needs). It is important to consider early on where the child's needs may be best met in order that the relevant people are involved early in discharge planning.

Fatigue is often a prominent feature in children following brain injury, and this will need to be considered when planning reintegration into school. It may be appropriate that graded return is considered or, in the older child, consideration paid to the ability to complete homework tasks within a given time – more time may be required.

Home adaptations

As well as adapting the school environment to a child's needs, an assessment will also need to be made of the child's home to ensure that participation and independence are promoted where possible. Access to the home, mobility around the home, and the ability to carry out activities of daily living, such as bathing and toileting, are part of this assessment.

Family life

A recent qualitative study looked at parents' experiences and support needs following childhood TBI, and found that parents had a number of unmet information and emotional support needs through the journey from the time of the injury to the child's return home. In particular, parents felt unsupported in managing their child's psychological needs and behaviour, and that there was a lack of information about ABI and potential future consequences of the injury [23].

Parents of children with less complex physical needs but ongoing cognitive and behavioural difficulties often find that it is more difficult to access support, particularly the brain injury has occurred many years beforehand.

SUMMARY

Children with ABI face many challenges following the initial injury and acute phase of recovery. Consequences of the brain injury may only emerge many years later as the child's developmental trajectory starts veering away from that of their peer group. Following brain injury, children often have particular difficulties with higher executive functions, skills which may only normally develop during adolescence.

Contrary to previous beliefs, children who suffer brain injury below the age of 3 years have poorer outcomes than older children following brain injury as their developmental trajectory is altered at a much earlier stage when neural pathways are forming.

There is little evidence in children with ABI to support the process of neurorehabilitation, particularly with regard to longer-term outcomes. However, functional outcomes have been shown to improve with early neurorehabilitation. It is important to develop a structured and goal-focussed approach with regular appraisal of these goals. The child and family should be central to this process.

Key points for clinical practice

- The earlier a brain injury in a child's development, the poorer the longer term prognosis.
- It is important to consider the longer term consequences of ABI as deficits may not be evident until many years after the injury.
- Rehabilitation should be a child and family centred approach and consist of goal-based interventions.

REFERENCES

1. Acker S, Ross J, Partrick D, et al. Glasgow motor score alone is equivalent to Glasgow Coma Scale at identifying children at risk for serious traumatic brain injury. J Trauma Acute Care Surg 2014; 77:304–309.
2. Phang I, Mathieson C, Sexton I, et al. Paediatric head injury admissions over a 10 year period in a regional neurosurgical unit. Scott Med J 2012; 57:152–156.
3. Billmire M, Myers P. Serious head injury in infants: accident or abuse? Pediatrics 1985; 75:340–342.
4. Thurman D. The epidemiology of traumatic brain injury in children and youths: a review of research since 1990. J Child Neurol 2014; pii: 0883073814544363 (Epub ahead of print).
5. Giza C, Hovda D. The new neurometabolic cascade of concussion. Neurosurgery 2014; 75:S24–S33.
6. Karver C, Wade S, Cassedy A, et al. Age at injury and long-term behaviour problems after traumatic brain injury in young children. Rehabil Psychol 2012; 57:256–265.
7. Azouvi P. Neuroimaging correlates of cognitive and functional outcome after traumatic brain injury. Curr Opin Neurol 2000; 13:665–669.
8. Shaklai S, Peretz R, Spasser R, et al. Long term functional outcome after moderate to severe paediatric traumatic brain injury. Brain Inj 2014; 28:915–921.

9.   Keightley M, Sinopoli K, Tator C. Is there evidence for neurodegenerative change following traumatic brain injury in children and youth? A scoping review. Front Hum Neurosci 2014; 8:139.
10. Wilde E, Chu Z, Bigler E, et al. Diffusion tensor imaging in the corpus callosum in children after moderate to severe traumatic brain injury. J Neurotrauma 2006; 23:1412–1426.
11. Tasker R. Changes in white matter late after severe traumatic brain injury in childhood. Dev Neurosci 2006; 28:302–308.
12. NHS England. NHS Standard Contract for Paediatric Neurosciences: Neurorehabilitation (2013/2014). Section B Part 1– Service specifications. Redditch: NHS England, 2013.
13. Tepas J, Leaphart C, Pieper P, et al. The effect of delay in rehabilitation on outcome of severe traumatic brain injury. J Paediatr Surg 2009; 44:368–372.
14. Kirk K, Shoykhet M, Jeong J, et al. Dysautonomia after pediatric brain injury. Dev Med Child Neurol 2012; 54:759–764.
15. Anderson V, Brown S, Newitt H, et al. Educational, vocational, psychosocial, and quality-of-life outcomes for adult survivors of childhood traumatic brain injury. J Head Trauma Rehabil 2009; 24:303–312.
16. Anderson V, Spencer-Smith M, Coleman L, et al. Predicting neurocognitive and behavioural outcome after early brain insult. Dev Med Child Neurol 2014; 56:329–336.
17. Anderson V, Eren S, Dob R, et al. Early attention impairment and recovery profiles after childhood traumatic brain injury. J Head Trauma Rehabil 2012; 27:199–209.
18. Ryan N, Anderson V, Godfrey C, et al. Predictors of very-long-term sociocognitive function after pediatric traumatic brain injury: evidence for the vulnerability of the immature "social brain". J Neurotrauma 2014; 31: 649–657.
19. Timonen M, Miettunen J, Hakko H, et al. The association of preceding traumatic brain injury with mental disorders, alcoholism and criminality: the Northern Finland 1966 Birth Cohort Study. Psychiatry Res 2002; 113: 217–226.
20. Hawley C. Self-esteem in children after traumatic brain injury: an exploratory study. NeuroRehabilitation 2012; 30:173–181.
21. World Health Organisation (WHO). International classification of functioning, disability and health (ICF). Geneva, Switzerland: WHO, 2001.
22. Steenbeck D, Marjolijn K, Galama K, et al. Goal attainment scaling in paediatric rehabilitation: a critical review of literature. Dev Med Child Neurol 2007; 49:550–556.
23. Kirk S, Fallon D, Fraser C, et al. Supporting parents following childhood traumatic brain injury: a qualitative study to examine information and emotional support needs across key care transitions. Child Care Health Dev 2015; 41:303–313.

Chapter 12

Neurotoxicity of agents used in paediatric anaesthesia

Hannah Gill

INTRODUCTION

Millions of fetuses, neonates and young children are exposed to anaesthetic drugs every year [1]. Two recent review articles cite numerous laboratory studies, which have shown that exposure of the developing brain to all commonly used anaesthetic drugs is associated with cell damage in the brain in a variety of immature mammals, including nonhuman primates [2,3]. To date, the published clinical studies of neurodevelopmental outcome after anaesthetic exposure have been retrospective and observational in design, and are unable to separate the anaesthetic exposure from the associated surgery [2,3]; therefore, they have been unable to provide definitive reassurance.

The concern is uppermost for the many children who unfortunately face multiple procedures or surgeries in their early life, predominantly due to premature birth. According to an expert group's report and statement on anaesthetic neurotoxicity and neuroplasticity, they 'recognised two critical factors determining anaesthetic neurotoxicity: the stage of brain development at the time of exposure and the degree of anaesthetic exposure, which includes both exposure frequency and cumulative anaesthetic dose' [4].

This chapter summarises the clinical and key preclinical evidence; outlines the difficulties faced in interpreting the results of these studies; and provides some guidance for the paediatrician asked by the parents of babies or young children to explain the risks associated with exposure to anaesthetic agents.

GENERAL ANAESTHESIA IS UNAVOIDABLE

In paediatric practice, sedation and anaesthesia are commonly indicated to facilitate necessary painful or distressing procedures. As early as 1987, Anand et al demonstrated, in a randomised control trial, the profound stress response in neonates not given fentanyl, undergoing patent ductus arteriosus ligation. [5] They found that neonates undergoing cardiac surgery and randomised to 'deeper anaesthesia' had better attenuation of stress responses and improved outcomes when compared to those randomised to 'lighter

Hannah Gill FRCA PhD, School of Physiology and Pharmacology, University of Bristol, Bristol, UK. Email: hannah.gill@bristol.ac.uk (for correspondence)

anaesthesia' [6]. The same group also demonstrated that neuronal activation and cell death in the brains of immature rats (subcortical or cortical areas dependent on the stage of maturation) following inflammatory pain had decreased cognitive function and increased pain thresholds in later life [7]. The cognitive effects were ameliorated by ketamine analgesia [7]. Other pre-clinical evidence has also shown that unopposed pain in the neonatal period produces adverse long-term neurodevelopmental outcomes such as hyperalgesia and neuroendocrine changes [2].

CLINICAL EVIDENCE

Published clinical studies of neuroanaesthetic toxicity to the developing brain have so far consisted of retrospective, observational, cohort or case–control studies, and recent updates have been covered in two excellent recent reviews [2,3]. These studies have suggested that there is an association between behavioural problems or developmental deficits and early exposure to anaesthesia, and that learning difficulties are more profound where multiple or prolonged exposures to anaesthesia have been experienced. However, it is impossible to separate the effect of anaesthesia from other factors such as inflammation, pain, stress or comorbidity, and these studies have also been confounded by a lack of detailed information about the perioperative physiology, postoperative care, specific drugs used and comorbidities [2,3].

One important reassuring study compared over 1000 monozygotic twin pairs in the Netherlands Twin Registry [8]. The parents reported exposure to anaesthesia before 3 years of age and between 3 and 12 years of age. At around 12 years of age, the educational achievement and occurrence of cognitive problems were assessed using standardised tests and ratings by the teachers of the children. Comparing the outcomes of pairs of twins where both were exposed to anaesthesia and pairs where neither were exposed to anaesthesia before the age of 3 showed that exposure to anaesthesia was associated with significantly lower educational achievement scores and significantly more cognitive problems. However, more importantly, outcomes of individuals from pairs of twins where one was exposed to anaesthesia and the other was not, in discordant twins, did not differ. Thus, there was no evidence for a causal relationship between anaesthesia exposure and later learning-related outcomes in this study.

However, another important more recent study has suggested that there is an association between a single surgical or diagnostic procedure requiring anaesthesia before 3 years of age and then deficits in language and abstract reasoning at 10 years of age [9]. The researchers used a prospectively collected Australian database originally created to investigate the long-term effects of perinatal ultrasound exposure. Out of almost 3000 children, only 9% were lost to follow-up by the age of 10 years and out of 11%, who were exposed to anaesthesia before the age of 3, 206 had a single exposure and 52 had multiple exposures. Neurocognitive testing evaluated expressive and receptive language ability, cognition, behaviour and motor function. After adjusting for confounders, a 2.4-fold increased risk for disabilities in receptive language when comparing children with a single exposure to those unexposed was found, and a 3.5-fold increased risk when comparing children with multiple exposures to those unexposed. Cognition testing revealed a 75% increased risk of disability in abstract reasoning in the single-exposure group versus the unexposed group, but no statistically significant difference when comparing those with multiple exposures. The other testing modalities did not differ between groups.

Bayesian meta-analysis involves formal combination of a prior distribution of a treatment effect, based on evidence not derived from the study under analysis, with a summary of the treatment effect from the data collected in the study, known as the likelihood, to yield an updated distribution of the quantity under analysis [10]. A Bayesian meta-analysis of paediatric anaesthesia and neurodevelopmental impairments, published in 2012, included English language publications presenting results comparing exposed and unexposed children <12 years of age and published after 2000 [11]. This analysis used 13 independent effect measures from 7 studies (including the 2 studies described above) and concluded that there was a 'modestly elevated risk of adverse behavioural or developmental outcomes in children who were exposed to anaesthesia and surgery during early childhood. The evidence, however, is considerably uncertain'. They state that the attributable risk of exposure to anaesthetic under 12 years of age in the United States is 2.6% (in contrast to 10.9% for cardiovascular disease from smoking) [11]. Bayesian methodology directly addresses the question of how new evidence should change what is currently believed and is controversial; in that it may involve the explicit use of subjective judgements in what is conventionally supposed to be a rigorous scientific exercise [10]. However, this metholodology is well suited to identifying potential future studies and this meta-analysis suggested that in future such a study will demonstrate a risk, even adjusted for multiple potentially confounding factors, with a probability of approximately 80%.

A collaboration between the US Food and Drug Administration and the International Anesthesia Research Society started a formal partnership, Strategies for Mitigating Anaesthesia-related Neurotoxicity in kids (SmartTots) and stated, in 2012, that the current evidence could not support a change in clinical practice. They are supporting, alongside basic sciences research, prospective clinical trials, which are currently underway.

Results from a pilot feasibility study for one of these trials, the Pediatric Anesthesia NeuroDevelopment Assessment (PANDA) project have been published [12]. The study aimed to address the two major challenges in using the proposed ambidirectional cohort design for the PANDA study, namely, retrospectively identifying and recruiting patients from a historical cohort and obtaining reliable clinical data related to anaesthesia exposure and surgery up to 10 years later. The proposed PANDA study protocol was successfully completed in 28 exposed–unexposed sibling pairs aged between 6 and 11 years, where the exposed siblings were American Society of Anesthesiologists' grade 1 or 2, i.e. healthy or with mild systemic disease. They had a single exposure to anaesthesia for inguinal hernia repair prior to 3 years of age and underwent direct testing using the Wechsler Abbreviated Scale of Intelligence and the NEuroPSYchological Assessment, second edition (NEPSY II). The parents completed questionnaires that related to behaviour using the Child Behaviour Checklist (CBCL) and Conners' parent rating scale. There were no differences between the two groups in T scores for any of the NEPSY II sub-domains, CBCL or Conners' scale. This trial is underway and aims to recruit 960 patients.

A Multi-site Randomized Controlled Trial Comparing Regional and General Anesthesia for Effects on Neurodevelopmental Outcome and Apnea in Infants (GAS) is an ongoing prospective, multinational, multicentre trial comparing several immediate postoperative physiologic variables including the incidence of apnoea and neurodevelopmental outcome at 2 and 5 years of age following inguinal hernia repair in neonates and infants born at 26 weeks' gestational age or greater and with postconceptual age of 60 weeks or less (NCT00756600) and has closed to recruitment with 722 participants. Unfortunately, presentation of the short-term primary outcome measures has already revealed significantly different cardiovascular physiological variables between the two groups.

Therefore, animal models will continue to be relied upon to better understand the mechanisms of toxicity and investigate potential therapeutic strategies.

PRECLINICAL EVIDENCE

Since the seminal work, at the beginning of this century, by Jevtovic-Todorovic et al showed an association between early exposure to midazolam, nitrous oxide and isoflurane (a clinically relevant combination of drugs) and widespread apoptotic neurodegeneration in the brains of neonatal rats, deficits in hippocampal synaptic function and persistent memory, and learning deficits [13], many studies investigating the phenomenon have been published. This drug-induced injury has been demonstrated in numerous immature rodent, and more recently, pig and nonhuman primate models.

The exposure of macaque monkeys in utero (on day 120 out of 165 days' gestation) to intravenous ketamine or propofol and early postnatal exposure [on postnatal (P) days 6–7] to isoflurane alone or in combination with nitrous oxide has been associated with widespread apoptosis and necrosis of cells in the brain and early postnatal exposure to ketamine has been associated with neurodevelopmental deficits [2,3]. Cell death after exposure was greater than twofold in the less mature animals and the pattern of damage, by brain regions, was different. Regarding duration of exposure, 3 hours of intravenous ketamine was not associated with increased apoptosis in two models, while 5 hours of ketamine or isoflurane was. While, as in clinical anaesthesia, control of physiological variables is possible in these models using invasive mechanical ventilation, pulse oximetry, and heart rate and blood pressure monitoring (noninvasive) the full-term macaque is considerably smaller than a term human (500 g versus 4000 g) and the optimal management of these models is very technically demanding. The plane of anaesthesia maintained in these macaques, despite being described as light by the authors, appears to be relatively deep; a surgical clamp was applied to the hand or foot every 30 minutes and the anaesthetic altered to maintain <10% change in the heart rate [14]. Exposure of newborn pigs, larger than macaques (by several kilograms) and where invasive blood pressure monitoring has been used, to isoflurane alone [15], and with nitrous oxide has also been associated with apoptosis after only 4 hours of anaesthesia [2,3].

However, by far the most preclinical evidence, from as early as 1993, has come from experimental models employing immature rodents. The literature is too extensive to discuss in depth here. In brief, these models have exposed fetal or immature rodents up to 3 weeks of age (an extreme preterm to small children human equivalent, depending on the anatomical site and developmental process that is compared [16]) to all the commonly used anaesthetic and sedative agents. Most, however, have utilised rodents in the first 2 weeks of life, during peak synaptogenesis, the period of vulnerability. Toxic effects have been demonstrated with all the commonly used anaesthetic drugs. Rodent studies have also assessed long-term functional outcomes and demonstrated association with exposure and impaired memory, and cognitive function. Interestingly, rodent studies have shown that an enriched environment reversed memory deficit in neonatal rodents after exposure to sevoflurane [17].

It is recognised that the durations of exposure and doses used in the rodent models have tended to be relatively prolonged and high; suppression of cardiopulmonary function leads to confounders with hypercarbia, respiratory distress and even mortality during exposure all reported. It is noteworthy in this setting that hypercarbia alone is associated with increased apoptosis in the developing brain of immature rodents [18]. However, worryingly, a single 1-hour exposure to the isoflurane at a dose lower than that required to produce an equivalent to surgical anaesthesia has been associated with apoptosis in the brain. Regional anaesthesia, a possible alternative to general anaesthesia, can unfortunately not be assumed to be free of toxicity; intrathecal administration of ketamine has been associated with increased apoptosis in the spinal cord of immature rats [19].

MECHANISMS OF ANAESTHESIA AND ANAESTHETIC-INDUCED NEUROAPOPTOSIS

In practice, general anaesthesia has numerous components: suppression of the response to painful stimulus (analgesia), immobility (muscle relaxation), and amnesia and hypnosis. These functional endpoints are usually achieved using multiple drugs, such as opiates, intravenous and inhalational anaesthetics, benzodiazepines and nonsteroidal anti-inflammatories rather than a single agent [20]. Alongside these drugs, in particular circumstances, neuromuscular blockade may be indicated to facilitate endotracheal intubation, mechanical ventilation or surgical access (e.g. laparotomy) and other drugs may be administered, such as anticoagulants and antibiotics. Clinical anaesthesia balances the maintenance of homeostasis with the avoidance of awareness and unnecessarily deep anaesthesia which would lead to prolonged recovery or postoperative side effects such as nausea. Where necessary, this balance is facilitated by using invasive ventilation and monitoring. Formal depth of anaesthesia monitoring with processed electroencephalography (EEG) is not routinely used in paediatric anaesthesia, and the close monitoring of vital signs and the end-tidal concentration of inhaled anaesthetic is relied upon.

The hypnotic effect of midazolam, propofol and the commonly used volatile inhalational anaesthetics (isoflurane, desflurane and sevoflurane) is thought, a least in part, to be the result of positive modulation of the inhibitory receptor γ-amino butyric acid type A (GABA-A) receptor, a neurotransmitter-gated chloride channel which reduces activation of mature neurones. The predominant effects of nitrous oxide, ketamine and xenon and some effects of isoflurane are the consequence of inhibitory action on the excitatory N-methyl-D-aspartate receptor. Neuroapoptosis (programmed cell death), the predominantly studied mechanism of anaesthetic-induced cell death, occurs during normal development, triggered by an extrinsic pathway (most important in immune cells) or an intrinsic pathway (where the mitochondria plays a key role) [1]. It was believed that failure to make synaptic connections and/or lack of neurotrophic support caused natural cell death in up to 50% of neurons during development, but newly developed methods for identifying and counting apoptotic profiles have shown that the majority of this cell death occurs in proliferating cell populations not yet differentiated into neurons [1]. It has been postulated that suppression of activity, as with anaesthesia, may render a neuron redundant and trigger apoptosis via the internal pathway [2]. All the volatile anaesthetics, propofol, ketamine, midazolam, nitrous oxide, thiopentone have been associated with increased apoptosis.

This evidence fits with the theory that unnecessarily deep anaesthesia is associated with poor outcomes; there is limited, and poorly understood, evidence from adult studies showing an association between poor outcome and deep anaesthesia, i.e. this association was independent of the dose given and therefore indicative of an individual's susceptibility to anaesthesia [21].

The patterns of electrocortical activity change during maturation and drugs used during anaesthesia differentially affect activity; some produce burst suppression pattern in the EEG at low dose, while others do not even at high dose [22]. In one human study of electrocortical activity in children aged from 9 days to 12 years, burst-like electrocortical activity was seen to persist from deep anaesthesia to emergence in all infants below 6 months of age, but not in children >1 year of age [23]. Two neonatal rodent studies have shown seizure-like activity in the EEG during isoflurane and sevoflurane exposure, more predominant in less mature rats and that this activity was associated with apoptosis in the brain [24,25]. This has led to the conclusion that toxicity was associated with seizure activity in developing brain rather than with unnecessarily deep anaesthesia. Interestingly, it has been shown that GABAergic cells may change polarity during development being excitatory earlier on before switching to inhibitory at around 7–10 days in the rat.

LIMITATIONS OF THE PRECLINICAL STUDIES

Translation across species from rodents to nonhuman primates and humans is confounded by interspecies differences in rates of maturation. An expert group on anaesthetic neurotoxicity and neuroplasticity noted that peak synaptogenesis does not occur at the same time in all brain regions, even within the same species [4]. While anaesthetic exposure of neonatal rats on postnatal day (P)7 was associated with histological damage in the thalamus, hippocampus and neocortex; on postnatal day 21 (P21), histological damage was seen in the dentate gyrus. Even within the same brain regions there are subgroups of susceptible cells. On P7, glutaminergic and GABAergic neurons are more susceptible than cholinergic neurons.

While this can be overcome by careful experimental design which focuses on specific brain regions and using large databases of comparisons of maturation across species, such as that found at www.translatingtime.com, comparison of dose across species and across different postnatal ages within species remains poorly understood. Assays comparing dose–response which rely on assessing responses to stimulation rely on equal maturations of both the sensory and motor processing, known to develop rapidly during postnatal development and very differently between species.

Studies using newborn pigs or nonhuman primates, where good control of physiological variables has been achieved, show a convincing association between clinically relevant anaesthetic exposures and neuroapoptosis. However, whether the doses used to simulate the clinical condition can be directly translated is debatable. It is notable that animals require higher doses of anaesthesia than humans [2] and that anaesthetic requirements appear to peak during the early postnatal period in rats, pigs and humans. However, this may not reflect a need for higher doses in early life or in less-developed species, but only the differential maturation of the nervous system on which judging of dosing relied.

Despite the criticisms, rodent models provide conditions to compare the effect of single agents or mixtures of drugs and generate potential strategies to be examined in larger animal and human studies. The future potential agent includes xenon, lithium and dexmedetomidine.

SUMMARY

Concerns regarding anaesthetic neurotoxicity in early life are not unfounded, but the evidence remains weak, and eagerly awaited prospective clinical studies may not provide definitive answers. A change in clinical practice has not yet been advised. However, surgeons are now more alert to the serious consideration of whether procedures in early life are warranted or could safely be delayed. Paediatricians using sedating drugs or referring to young children for sedation should also consider this. However, this always needs to be balanced with the risks of unopposed pain in early life.

Further information for clinicians and families can be found on the internet at: www. apagbi.org.uk and www.smarttots.org.

Key points for clinical practice

- Numerous laboratory studies have shown that exposure of the developing brain to all commonly used anaesthetic and sedative drugs is associated with cell damage.
- Millions of fetuses, neonates and young children are exposed to anaesthetic drugs every year and the concern about toxicity is uppermost for the those requiring multiple procedures or surgeries in early life.
- Clinical studies of neuroanaesthetic toxicity in the developing brain have so far consisted of retrospective, observational studies providing weak evidence and do not support a change in clinical practice.
- Prospective clinical trials are underway and will report in several years.
- Clinicians caring for children need to be able to inform and reassure worried parents and be able to weigh up the risks of delaying procedures which result in exposure to these drugs.
- Information for clinicians and families is available online.

REFERENCES

1. Creeley CE, Olney JW. The young: neuroapoptosis induced by anesthetics and what to do about it. Anesth Analg 2010; 110:442–448.
2. Sanders RD, Hassell J, Davidson AJ, et. al. Impact of anaesthetics and surgery on neurodevelopment: an update. Br J Anaesth 2013; 110:i53–i72.
3. Olsen EA, Brambrink AM. Anesthetic neurotoxicity in the newborn and infant. Curr Opin Anaesthesiol 2013; 26:535–542.
4. Jevtovic-Todorovic V, Absalom AR, Blomgren K, et al. Anaesthetic neurotoxicity and neuroplasticity: an expert group report and statement based on the BJA Salzburg Seminar. Br J Anaesth 2013; 111:143–151.
5. Anand KJ, Sippell WG, Aynsley-Green A. Randomised trial of fentanyl anaesthesia in preterm babies undergoing surgery: effects on the stress response. Lancet 1987; 1:243–248.
6. Anand KJ, Hickey PR. Halothane-morphine compared with high-dose sufentanil for anesthesia and postoperative analgesia in neonatal cardiac surgery. N Engl J Med 1992; 326:1–9.
7. Anand KJ, Garg S, Rovnaghi CR, et al. Ketamine reduces the cell death following inflammatory pain in newborn rat brain. Pediatr Res 2007; 62:283–290.
8. Bartels M, Althoff RR, Boomsma DI. Anesthesia and cognitive performance in children: no evidence for a causal relationship. Twin Res Hum Genet 2009; 12:246–253.
9. Ing C, DiMaggio C, Whitehouse A, et al. Long-term differences in language and cognitive function after childhood exposure to anesthesia. Pediatrics 2012; 130:e476–e485.
10. Spiegelhalter DJ, Myles JP, Jones DR, et al. Bayesian methods in health technology assessment: a review. Health Technol Assess 2000; 4:1–130.
11. DiMaggio C, Sun LS, Ing C, et al. Pediatric anesthesia and neurodevelopmental impairments: a Bayesian meta-analysis. J Neurosurg Anesthesiol 2012; 24:376–381.
12. Sun LS, Li G, DiMaggio CJ, et al. Feasibility and pilot study of the Pediatric Anesthesia NeuroDevelopment Assessment (PANDA) project. J Neurosurg Anesthesiol 2012; 24:382–388.
13. Jevtovic-Todorovic V, Hartman RE, Izumi Y, et al. Early exposure to common anesthetic agents causes widespread neurodegeneration in the developing rat brain and persistent learning deficits. J Neurosci 2003; 23:876–882.

14. Brambrink AM, Evers AS, Avidan MS, et al. Isoflurane-induced neuroapoptosis in the neonatal rhesus macaque brain. Anesthesiology 2010; 112:834–841.

15. Sabir H, Bishop S, Cohen N, et al. Neither xenon nor fentanyl induces neuroapoptosis in the newborn pig brain. Anesthesiology 2013; 119:345–357.

16. Workman AD, Charvet CJ, Clancy B, et al. Modeling transformations of neurodevelopmental sequences across mammalian species. J Neurosci 2013; 33:7368–7383.

17. Shih J, May LD, Gonzalez HE, et al. Delayed environmental enrichment reverses sevoflurane-induced memory impairment in rats. Anesthesiology 2012; 116:586–602.

18. Stratmann G, May LD, Sall JW, et al. Effect of hypercarbia and isoflurane on brain cell death and neurocognitive dysfunction in 7-day-old rats. Anesthesiology 2009; 110:849–861.

19. Walker SM, Westin BD, Deumens R, et al. Effects of intrathecal ketamine in the neonatal rat: evaluation of apoptosis and long-term functional outcome. Anesthesiology 2010; 113:147–159.

20. Urban BW, Bleckwenn M. Concepts and correlations relevant to general anaesthesia. Br J Anaesth. 2002; 89:3–16.

21. Monk TG, Weldon BC. Anesthetic depth is a predictor of mortality: it's time to take the next step. Anesthesiology 2010; 112:1070–1072.

22. Murrell JC, Waters D, Johnson CB. Comparative effects of halothane, isoflurane, sevoflurane and desflurane on the electroencephalogram of the rat. Lab Anim 2008; 42:161–170.

23. Davidson AJ, Sale SM, Wong C, et al. The electroencephalograph during anesthesia and emergence in infants and children. Paediatr Anaesth 2008; 18:60–70.

24. Edwards DA, Shah HP, Cao W, et al. Bumetanide alleviates epileptogenic and neurotoxic effects of sevoflurane in neonatal rat brain. Anesthesiology 2010; 112:567–575.

25. Seubert CN, Zhu W, Pavlinec C, et al. Developmental effects of neonatal isoflurane and sevoflurane exposure in rats. Anesthesiology 2013; 119:358–364.

Index

Note: Page numbers in **bold** or *italic* refer to tables or figures, respectively.